THE
ITIS
REVEALED

By

Curtis H. Price

Published by Curtis H. Price

Cover design by Curtis H. Price

ISBN-13: 979-8-218-24683-9

For speaking engagements and bulk book orders:

Websites:
www.curtispricelive.com
www.theitisrevealed.com
www.fraternalfitness.com

Instagram and YouTube:
@curtispricelive

DEDICATION

To my grandmother, Maria B. Lowe, for always telling me I could, and for those throughout my life who told me I couldn't. Thank you.

ACKNOWLEDGMENTS

To my amazing wife Paula and two children
Laila and Aaron, I love you, and thank you
for always being my biggest supporters!

TABLE OF CONTENTS

HELLO!

First, I want to thank you for selecting this book. Second, I want to congratulate you on taking a major step toward living a healthier lifestyle. Before we get started, I'd like to take a moment to introduce myself and give you some background information that will help you understand why I am writing about health in the first place.

I have always been comfortable talking to people from all walks of life about health, regardless of their religion, beliefs, nationality, or ethnicity. I was born in Heidelberg, Germany, and traveled throughout Europe and the Caribbean during my youth and into my teenage years. I was exposed to many cultures and witnessed how their lifestyles were often different than most Americans. While living in Europe and traveling to many countries, so many people relied on walking and biking as a primary means of transportation. Food was often purchased at local markets, farms, or shops. Meats always came from a butcher, and even wines were purchased from a local vineyard. The idea of sourcing locally was very familiar to me at a young age. Fresh foods and exercise were always a way of life.

During my time growing up, my household was not typical. I was heavily influenced by my grandparents who were true pioneers and way ahead of their time. In 1971, they opened Laurel Health Foods Inc., which was one of the, if not *the*, first health food stores located between Washington, DC, and Baltimore, Maryland. By no means was this an easy task. People poked fun and made jokes about them selling and using vitamins. However, they were very determined and hardworking and never wavered in their belief that fresh, whole foods and vitamins should be accessible to anyone. At this time, the concept of a large-scale grocery store dedicated to fresh, whole foods and vitamins did not exist. It was not until the early '90s that you could find a chain grocery store fully dedicated to natural and organic foods, vitamins, and cosmetics, as there were not enough products on the market nor was there enough consumer demand.

Fast forward forty-five years, and Laurel Health Food Inc. is still a family owned and operated business that focuses on providing high-quality supplements to deliver overall health benefits for people of all ages and backgrounds.

I always chuckle when I think back to the plate—yes, plate—of vitamins that I would have to take before heading to school. If you think we were eating

Frosted Flakes or Fruity Pebbles or any of those sugar-laden, artificially colored cereals for breakfast, you are wrong and have grossly misjudged my grandparents. My brother and I would always attempt to make a strong case about the cool kids in the cereal commercials, but there was no winning that debate. I remember when tofu emerged on the health food scene. It was weirdly packaged: it came in a rectangular, plastic container with water surrounding a large white block. The labels would never stick, and we never had seen anything that looked like this that we wanted to eat! And because we were kids, we had all kinds of jokes about anything with a name remotely close to *foot* or *toe*. My brother and I would also work at the health food store after school and during the summer where my grandfather would always instruct us to "straighten up the merchandise on the shelves" Their commitment to health influenced my life, my parenting, and, subsequently, my children's diet. Looking back, I am so thankful that my upbringing had such a strong health and wellness component.

Once I finished middle school, my family moved to Vicenza, Italy, where I attended high school. While in Vicenza, I started getting into the gym for sports and, more importantly, for the girls! I always wanted to pump iron and get ripped. At this time, I was much more interested in discovering new protein powders and amino acids. As a young man whose family owned a health food store, I had access to try almost any protein powder or supplement that any of the different vendors and/or manufacturers carried. Reluctantly, I would drink tons of various nasty protein drink concoctions. Due to my growing interest in sports and physical fitness, I started to pay more attention to the types of supplements that I could take to help with my weightlifting endeavors. Even then, there was still a relatively limited number of products to try, but you could see an increase in new merchandise coming to the market. After discovering my newfound interests, visiting my grandparent's health food store every summer took on a different meaning. With this influx of new products landing in our health food store, my grandfather would make sure we "straightened up" the merchandise, and he expected us to pitch in with all aspects of the store while visiting!

Once I finished high school, I attended college and graduated from Bowie State University in 1999. While at Bowie State University, I played on the intramural soccer team, was an ROTC cadet, and kept working out. I always had vitamins in my dorm room and various "health food" snacks. Now, here is a real gem of advice for anyone heading off to college: buy organic or healthy "munchies." When your friends visit your dorm room sniffing for a late-night snack and they see anything that looks remotely "healthy," they'll do a 180° and head in the other direction! Trust me, I loved telling them that my cookies were from a health food store and that they probably wouldn't find them appetizing.

Aside from dealing with the late-night snack raiders, something else was starting to happen. I began taking on the role of a quasi-health advisor. Fellow classmates would come up to me and ask what natural remedy they should use for a cold. They also sought my advice about taking vitamins and other supplements. I never really paid that much attention to these inquiries. I would make my suggestion and not think too much about it after giving the advice. During the winter months at the university, many of my friends would come down with a cold. I would recommend and often give various supplements that I used to help boost my immune system and help combat the latest cold passing through campus.

After graduating with a Bachelor of Science in Business Administration with a Marketing concentration, I pursued various jobs within this field. However, I ended up being drawn back to my family's health food store. I then began to take on a more serious role in the business: I started to help manage the family store. I got more involved with the daily operations, sourcing and ordering the packaged foods as well as locating new vendors and other products to add to the store inventory. It was around this time that Dr. Robert Atkins came out with Advantage Meal Replacement Bars. We carried and sold all kinds of bars, but by no means were people walking out with two to eight boxes of bars like they did with the Atkins bars. Being the marketing guy that I am, I became very interested in why these bars sold so well and, more importantly, if there were any other products like them on the market.

Atkins brand products and other weight loss products from different companies started to fill the shelves in the early 2000s. What had been one shelf for low-carb products became an entire section of low-carb products. I then started to track the sales of this section and decided that I could open a specialty store that sold nothing but low-carbohydrate and low-sugar products. You would have thought I was a deranged lunatic with the feedback I received when I first started telling friends and family about my low-carb store idea. The only person, excluding my partner who happened to be my younger brother, that encouraged me to go for it was my mom.

On July 15, 2003, I opened the first low-carbohydrate and low-sugar store in the DC, Maryland, and Virginia area called Whoa . . . That's Lo! LLC. We felt like pioneers of the low-carb frontier! Before we opened for business, I did extensive reading and research and was somewhat obsessed with learning as much as I could about the Dr. Atkins diet. I began to pay more attention to what I was consuming. The opening of this store marked one of the most definitive points in my life when I began to truly understand the impact sugar and refined carbohydrates had on my health and the health of others.

I began researching and reading anything I could on health as it related to sugar and the food industry. One book in particular, *Sweetness and Power* by Sidney W. Mintz, tracks sugar's role throughout history in relation to slavery. Mintz paints the picture that connects slavery and sugar:

> *Sugar cane was first carried to the New World by Columbus on his second voyage, in 1493; he brought it there from the Spanish Canary Islands. Cane was first grown in the New World in Spanish Santo Domingo; it was from that point that sugar was first shipped back to Europe, beginning around 1516. Santo Domingo's pristine sugar industry was worked by enslaved Africans, the first slaves having been imported there soon after the sugar cane. Hence it was Spain that pioneered sugar cane, sugar making, African slave labor, and the plantation form in the Americas.* (1)

After reading Mintz, I gained more of an understanding of how sugar, as a commodity, influenced history, the slave trade, and industry. Another great author that changed my entire viewpoint of health, especially around natural food products, is Doug. A. Kaufmann, author of *Fungus Link, Fungus Link 2*, and *Infectious Diabetes*. Kaufmann was so profound because he illustrated the true culprit of people's

addiction to consuming high-sugar and high-carbo-
hydrate foods by identifying the culprit as a fungus:

> We *don't* read about the studies of twins who
> have grown up apart. In those studies, though
> they certainly still appear *identical,* each twin's
> medical history demonstrates a *different* suscep-
> tibility to disease. That's just one example from a
> growing bank of evidence that, with regard to
> health, the *habits we learn* from our parents often
> carry more weight than the *genes we inherit.* (2)

During this period, my Friday night happy hours
at TGIF started to change. I began looking differently
at menu options. For example, I would replace french
fries for broccoli with my chicken tenders as well as
order a diet soda versus a regular soda. This may not
read as the healthiest meal, but it marked the start of
a new food consciousness. I always understood the
value of eating whole, fresh foods because of my upbringing. However, during this time as a young, single
man, I was not the best cook, and I did not always
have access to fresh, home-cooked meals. But I realized that I could take charge of what I chose to put in
my body. À la carte options and "skinny" menus did
not exist back then, so I began to customize my meals
while eating out. I found myself reading health books
at happy hour instead of watching sports or talking
to other people. I was consumed. But I must admit
that I met more women reading at happy hour than I
ever had in the past! After opening Whoa . . . That's

Lo!, I could not in good conscience sell or promote something that I did not practice and believe in!

Much to everyone's amazement, the store was a huge success. Low-carb living took the country by storm. It was in the news back then more than the Kardashians are now. When we first opened Whoa . . . That's Lo!, my father would make periodic visits to see what type of venture his two boys had gotten themselves into. To my amazement, one day I witnessed him turning a package of cheesecake over to check the nutritional labels. He was checking the sugar content on various items we carried to see if he could eat them himself. My father is a type 2 diabetic, and when he said that a certain low-carb product was sugar-free and safe for him to eat, I saw the potential these products had in helping diabetics. At that moment, a light went on and changed my perception of low-carb foods forever. So many people were focused on losing X number of pounds on the Atkins diet that they didn't realize the huge benefits these foods had in fighting diabetes. Alas, not long after, the country's love affair with the low-carb diet craze came to a swift halt. The bottom of the industry literally seemed to fall out from under our feet. Sales took a nosedive, and the "fad" was over—or so we all thought. The store eventually closed, and we merged our various products into the family health food store in Laurel, MD.

In 2010, I founded CrossFit Laurel and fully began to implement healthy living into my community. Right before the store closed, I was researching various physical training methodologies that I could incorporate into a fitness routine. I found the Crossfit website, and I admit, I did not fully understand the various workout programs on this site. However, I was blown away by the focus given to nutrition and how it pertained to sugar. I always found it ironic when I saw an overweight personal trainer or health professional. I believe if you're not remotely fit or healthy, why in the world should people listen to you about fitness? Since I believed in practicing what you preach, I wanted to focus not only on food consumption but also on the quality of my physical activity. CrossFit harmoniously blended my two worlds of health and physical fitness.

I am writing this book to shed light on what I perceive to be a very simple problem, which has become so complex due to the increasing number of so-called experts and health professionals in these fields. I feel there is an abundance of books on the market today that are full of just "stuff." I was recently in a bookstore and was amazed at the number of various quick-fix books on the shelves. Topics varied from twenty-eight-day detoxes to losing weight by drinking broth. Further, many health and weight loss publications seem to be written by doctors for doctors. Due to the complexity of the information given, having a medical dictionary by your side to truly understand the content seems necessary. Wading through an ocean of technical terms and trying to decipher the information can be an exhausting task.

However, even with the abundance of information that has been published about health and wellness, we still have escalating populations of people being diagnosed with diabetes and obesity. Even more saddening are the numbers of children being diagnosed with *adult* health problems. This is why it was important to me to write a book that not only spells out what you should eat and how you can live a truly healthy lifestyle in layman's terms, but also discusses one of the most addictive and destructive drugs known to man that has infiltrated our diet throughout recorded history: SUGAR! With that said, I give you *The Itis Revealed.*

CHAPTER 1

SUGAR'S ROLE
IN HISTORY

○●○

To provide insight into sugar's emergence in the world, I've noted key periods in time significant to the role of sugar's popularity today. It is important to note that some of these dates are before the start of the channeled slavery to the Americas. This begins to outline sugar's emergence onto the global scene and illustrates its deep-seated roots in history and the impact that it had on civilizations. (1,2,3,4,5,6,7,8,9)

SUGAR's ROLE IN HISTORY

PRE 510 BC SUGAR IS FIRST USED IN POLYNESIA. **510 BC** PERSIAN EMPEROR DARIUS, AFTER INVADING INDIA, DISCOVERS SUGAR CANE.

642 BC ARABS INVADE PERSIA, FIND SUGAR CANE AND BEGIN PRODUCTION IN THEIR EXPANDING TERRITORIES.

11TH CENTURY AD EUROPEANS DISCOVER SUGAR DURING THE CRUSADES.

1492 COLUMBUS SAILS THE OCEAN BLUE AND FINDS THE AMERICAS. **1493** COLUMBUS BRINGS SUGAR CANE PLANT TO GROW IN CARIBBEAN.

1502 IMPORTATION OF AFRICAN SLAVES TO THE CARIBBEAN BEGIN.

MID 16TH CENTURY THE PORTUGUESE IN BRAZIL SWITCH FROM DEVELOPING THE BRAZIL WOOD TRADE TO SUGAR CANE PRODUCTION AND BEGIN TO IMPORT AFRICAN SLAVES.

1619 LATE AUGUST THE 1ST AFRICAN ARRIVES IN VIRGINIA. **1620 NOVEMBER 11TH** PILGRIMS ARRIVE ON PLYMOUTH ROCK VIA THE MAYFLOWER.

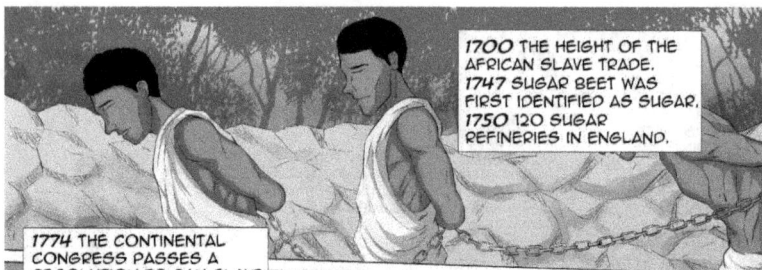

1700 THE HEIGHT OF THE AFRICAN SLAVE TRADE. **1747** SUGAR BEET WAS FIRST IDENTIFIED AS SUGAR. **1750** 120 SUGAR REFINERIES IN ENGLAND.

1774 THE CONTINENTAL CONGRESS PASSES A RESOLUTION TO BAN SLAVE IMPORTATION. **1808** THE IMPORTATION OF SLAVES INTO U.S. WAS BANNED AND PROHIBITED AMERICANS FROM ENGAGING IN THE TRADE.

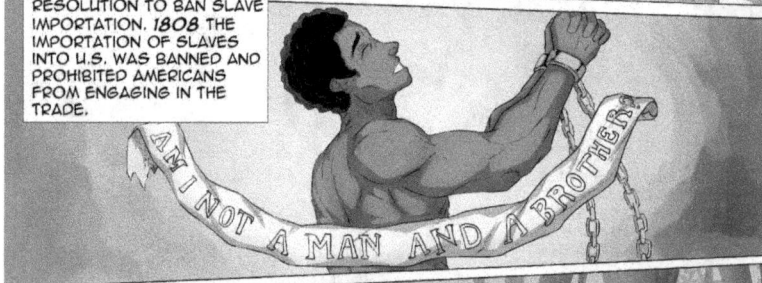

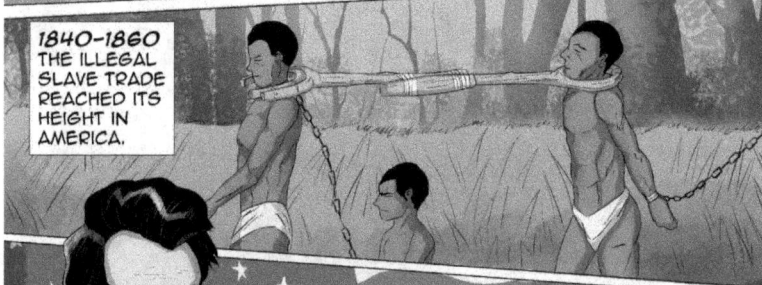

AM I NOT A MAN AND A BROTHER

1840–1860 THE ILLEGAL SLAVE TRADE REACHED ITS HEIGHT IN AMERICA.

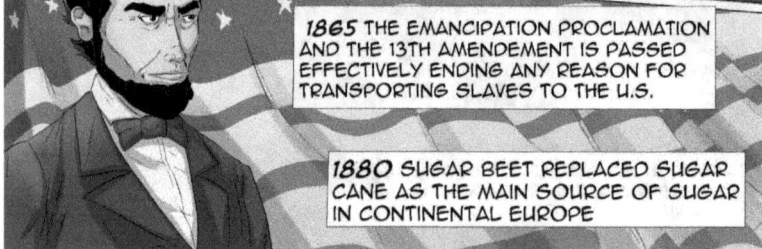

1865 THE EMANCIPATION PROCLAMATION AND THE 13TH AMENDEMENT IS PASSED EFFECTIVELY ENDING ANY REASON FOR TRANSPORTING SLAVES TO THE U.S.

1880 SUGAR BEET REPLACED SUGAR CANE AS THE MAIN SOURCE OF SUGAR IN CONTINENTAL EUROPE

From the beginning of this timeline, major battles were fought. Sugar was discovered by the victor of the battle and brought it back to their land to cultivate. This pattern was repeated in subsequent battles where the same chain of events took place. The Crusades mark the defining period in history where Europe was introduced to sugar as a luxury. Royalty was the only privileged class even to experience the taste of sugar.

Over generations, sugar remained a luxury of royalty, and few commoners ever had the chance to taste this newly discovered luxury. A German traveler in the sixteenth century, who met Queen Elizabeth at court, wrote, "The queen, in the 65th year of her age (as we were told), very majestic; her face oblong, fair but wrinkled; her eyes small, yet black and pleasant; her nose a little hooked, her lips narrow, and her teeth black (a defect the English seem subject to, from their too great use of sugar)." (10) This traveler observed that the poor in England looked healthier than the rich due to the fact that they could not afford and, in turn, consume such high amounts of sugar. (11)

These images paint a very different picture than what we're accustomed to in the movies and on television shows. These depictions of royalty are normally that they are attractive people leisurely strolling through the royal gardens with no apparent concerns for degenerating oral hygiene. Having a mouth full of black teeth paints a slightly different picture.

It is interesting to note that in modern society, the mentality about sugar consumption, for many, is opposite the mentality of what sugar historically represented. As previously illustrated, the royal elite, who were clearly more financially stable, did not understand the connection between health and certain foods. Today, more "elite" grocery retailers, such as specialty supermarkets and boutique grocery stores and chains, cater to shoppers in a higher income bracket. Yet even though "healthy shoppers" choose "organic" grocery stores, not all food choices available in these stores are healthy. And to compound the problem, people facing financial hardship may not be able to frequent high-end grocery stores where organic, "healthier" foods are available. The consumption of lower-quality, cheaper foods, such as dollar menus at fast-food traps set up on almost every highly traveled street corner in America, is fueling the health epidemic of obesity that we currently face as a nation. It is ironic that what was once only for the royal elite is now available to the masses. My goal is not only to bring awareness to healthy lifestyle habits but also, more importantly, to show people how they can empower themselves by turning these habits into a lifestyle.

Sugar wasn't always considered evil. During the early 1700s, there were well-respected doctors that supported unlimited sugar consumption. An Englishman by the name of Dr. Frederick Slare found sugar to be almost a cure-all. The only downfall was that the sugar, apparently, made the ladies too fat. During the seventeenth century, high consumption of sugar was already recognized as a cause of excess weight gain. In 1715, Dr. Slare wrote a book titled *A Vindication of Sugars Against the Charge of Dr. Willis, Other Physicians, and Common Prejudices: Dedicated to the Ladies.* For all you ladies, the good doctor wrote a special book just for you saying that sugar was not the culprit, even though I imagine he knew the consumption of sugar could lead to larger waistlines. (12)

Dr. Slare wrote this book in direct response to Dr. Willis and other physicians who opposed sugar. If you are not familiar with Dr. Willis, it is important to note his significant contribution to modern medicine. He added the term *mellitus*, which means "honey sweet," to the disease *diabetes*. (13) *Diabetes mellitus* was a separate designation for the disease. This was discovered when Dr. Willis noted that the urine of a diabetic had a sweet taste. Interestingly, three thousand years ago clinical features of this disease were described by ancient Egyptians, and the actual term *diabetes* was first coined by Aretaeus of Cappodocia (81–133 AD). (14) Many ancient societies (Greek, Chinese, Indian, and Persian) recorded their findings as they pertained to sweet-tasting urine. (15)

"English economic historian D.C. Coleman believes, per capita, consumption of sugar rose more rapidly than bread, meat, and dairy consumption between 1650 and 1750." (16) From 1650 to 1750, there was a spike in sugar consumption primarily due to the increased slave trade which made the availability of sugar more common for people of all classes. Mintz references Deerr in his estimation of British per-capita annual consumption of sugar between 1700 and 1800. (17)

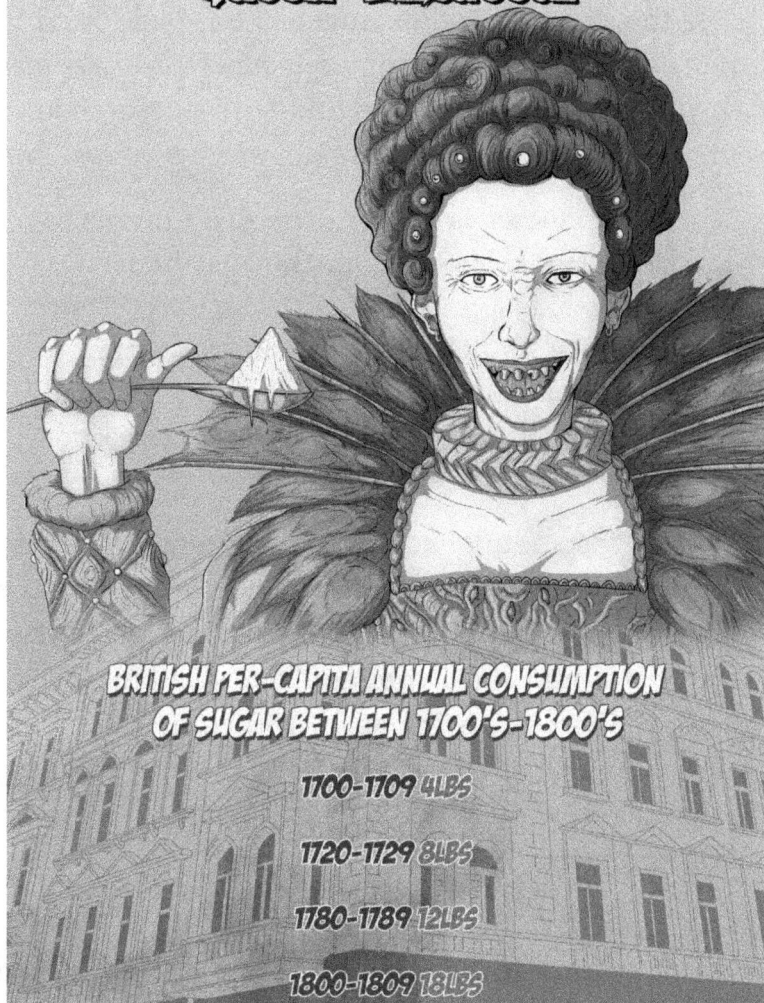

Queen Elizabeth

BRITISH PER-CAPITA ANNUAL CONSUMPTION
OF SUGAR BETWEEN 1700'S-1800'S

1700-1709 4LBS

1720-1729 8LBS

1780-1789 12LBS

1800-1809 18LBS

As we entered the 1800s, there was a drastic shift in sugar's status. At one time, sugar was a luxury of kings. Now, it had started to become a common luxury for the masses. Today, sugar is an item found in almost every food we consume. Around 1800, factory work was quickly on the rise, and both parents found themselves in the workforce:

> When the mother is at work there is no time to prepare porridge or broth in the 'diet hour' . . . usually breakfast and dinner become bread and butter meals. As the school interval for dinner is not the same as the mill 'diet hour' the children have to unlock the house and get 'pieces' for themselves. (18)

What's fascinating about that statement is that even during the 1800s, families were experiencing the same challenges with meals that we often face today. One never would have thought about latchkey kids walking the streets in the early 1800s, just like kids do today. With both parents often in the workforce, children fend for themselves when it comes to snacks and other meals.

In the 1870s, a condiment we take for granted—jam—started to become a very important factor in the diets of the working class. At this time, bread was a staple source of calories. However, due to the lack of modern-day preservatives, bread could quickly become stale. Smearing on a fruit spread was a tasty option when you had to eat hard, stale bread. Many fruit spreads were made as a way to preserve rotting fruit since sugar is an excellent preservative. In each case, something that would have been undesirable, (rotting fruit and stale bread), took on a new life. "Jam contains 50 to 65 percent of its weight in sugar." (19) Jam's high sugar content makes it a condiment that contributes to the expanding waistline of modern society.

In 1905, jam manufacturers agreed that their most lucrative market was the working class. Jam became a necessity and a substitute for the more expensive butter. (20) Hard-working people used jam as an essential source of calories. These days, we have seen an increase in not only the total consumption of sugar but also in the population of the middle and lower working classes. Once a luxury, sugar is now considered a daily staple to feed the demands of an ever-growing, labor-intensive working population. Today, as the middle class is slowly shrinking, the temptation for these families and individuals to consume less expensive, sugar-laden foods presents an increased threat to their health. In this modern age of information and technology where we have robotic vehicles on Mars and information literally at our fingertips, we still are burdened with issues leading to obesity and unhealthy lifestyles.

CHAPTER 2

IS SOUL FOOD REALLY FOOD FOR THE SOUL?

○●○

Looking back on my own personal experiences with soul food, I can still recall my great-grandma, Bennie, cooking with lard in her cozy little country home in Ridgeway, Virginia. Ridgeway is near Martinsville and is about two hours south of Richmond. There, I experienced my first taste of pig intestines, (more commonly known as chitterlings), a staple dish in traditional soul food. Foods like chitterlings are considered "scrap foods" and contributed to a sizable portion of the slaves nutritional requirements. Slaves also had the advantage of not having access to the more processed foods that their masters regularly ate, such as desserts that were made with processed sugar.

This early soul food, unlike the later iterations that contained more fried and sugary recipes, was void of sugar and processed carbohydrates, and it was not completely nutritionally deficient, in theory. The term *soul food* is often misleading. Often these foods are not necessarily positive, nutritionally speaking, for the body. However, these foods provide comfort because they conjure up memories often associated with family and times past. Though many African Americans today do not have direct ties to their ancestors, these foods connect them to their roots. The good news is we can look at some of the common dishes associated with soul food and extract from them the good and healthy components—so we can learn to avoid the *itis*.

What is this *itis*? This is a term that has been lovingly used in the African American vernacular for years. Even though the term may be new to some, the actual experience has been felt by most humans in history at least once in their lives. If you have ever overindulged on a meal and found yourself nodding off at the dinner table or wobbling around to find a comfortable area to rest for a moment, you have experienced the *itis*. Many foods that are popular in the African American community have contributed to countless episodes of the *itis*. Listed below are foods that emerged due to slavery and have been celebrated within various African American communities.

1. Shrimp and Grits (Creole Coast)

Grits originated from the Native American Muskogee tribe's preparation of Indian corn, similar to hominy. Traditionally from the Southeastern woodlands, the Muskogee would grind the corn in a stone mill, giving it the gritty texture that we are all familiar with. From this tribe, the preparation was passed down to settlers in the area because hominy was used as a form of currency. There are also known writings from the Gullah Geechee, descendants of slaves from West Africa, that mention meals resembling shrimp and grits. (1) This is most likely because the Gullah slaves would periodically receive allowance or food, including grits. Making the most of their local resources on the coast, the Gullahs would catch shrimp and other fish in nets and cook them in a variety of ways, including with grits. Since then, shrimp and grits have remained a breakfast dish found mainly in the low country marshes near the southern coast.

2. Hush Puppies

Hush puppies are derived from cornbread. It is said that hush puppies originated during the Civil War (1861–1865) when soldiers would throw fried cornbread to their dogs—to "hush the puppies." (2)

3. Collard Greens

Collard greens date back to prehistoric times and are one of the oldest members of the cabbage family. Collard greens are an extremely nutritious cool-season vegetable—rich in vitamins and minerals that help prevent and fight disease. Today, many varieties of greens—collards, mustard, turnips, chard, spinach, and kale—continue to be a traditional offering at picnics, potlucks, parties, and family dinners. (3) They are a staple in African American culture.

4. Molasses Water

Blackstrap molasses is a byproduct of sugar cane's refining process. Sugar cane is mashed to create juice and then boiled once to create cane syrup. A second boiling creates molasses. Blackstrap molasses contains vital vitamins and minerals, such as iron, calcium, magnesium, vitamin B6, and selenium. (4)

5. Sweet Potato Pie

Sweet potatoes and yams have been a large part of African Americans' diet since African slaves brought them to the United States in the 1600s. (5)

6. Red Beans and Rice

Red beans and rice is another traditional dish, especially in the Southern states. Red beans and rice is an emblematic dish of Louisiana Creole cuisine traditionally made on Mondays with red beans, vegetables, spices, and pork bones left over from Sunday dinner, cooked together slowly in a pot, and served over rice. (6)

7. Baked Macaroni and Cheese

Baked macaroni and cheese is a dish that African Americans introduced to the USA for breakfast on Christmas. (7)

8. Kwanzaa Brownies

Many African Americans celebrate Kwanzaa, a non-religious cultural holiday, from December 26 through January 1. During the seven days of Kwanzaa (which is derived from a Swahili word for "first fruits of the harvest"), African Americans celebrate their heritage and take pride in their African traditions. The Kwanzaa celebration was created by Dr. Maulana Karenga, an activist and scholar, who has been involved in the development of black studies and African

American art and student movements in the United States.

Each of the seven days of Kwanzaa represents a different principle, such as unity, purpose, and creativity. African American families celebrate this community-building holiday in their own way, with music, get-togethers, and feasting on brownies decorated with red, black, and green frosting made especially for these events. (8)

9. Hoppin' John

Hoppin' John is considered a dish for good luck. With both rice and black-eyed peas available, the natives of West Africa could prepare a dish that reminded them of home: a humble combination of rice and beans that became a widespread tradition. (9)

10. Cala Cake

Cala is known as a sweet-tasting rice cake. It was often served in the morning with café au lait and was sold by black women in the French Quarter of New Orleans. In the state of Georgia, the sweetened rice cake was called *saraka*. (10)

11. Guinea Corn

Guinea corn is also known as *sorghum* and *millet*. It was transported to the United States by Africans.

Guinea corn was used by Africans to make bread. It was also used to feed the fowl. (11)

12. Akarajé

In both Brazil and West Africa, *akarajé* is considered street food. Brazilians call it *akarajé*, and in West Africa, it is called *akara*, but it's the same meal made of black-eyed peas. These peas originated in Africa and were brought to America just like rice and gumbo. Americans serve it the same way too: with a crispy little beignet accompanied by some very hot sauce. (12)

13. Juba

Juba is a traditional slave food. The words *juba, jibba,* or *jiba* refer to the food that enslaved Africans working in the plantation house collected from the "massa's" leftovers. In this dish, all the leftovers were just mixed together. There was no way to distinguish the bread from the vegetables or meat. It was often shared with the field workers. (13)

Soul food has been used to describe a certain combination of food selections that primarily developed out of necessity by enslaved Africans. This connection between slavery and the prevalence of these key foods in modern society is undeniable. Enslaved Africans lived under grueling circumstances and endured extremely harsh conditions where they were forced into performing back-breaking, arduous labor. Being unwillingly torn from their homeland, Africans found comfort in their food and relied on various food traditions to survive. Slaves were fed leftovers or "scraps" from the slave owner's house. These foods were mostly pork-based, fried, and cooked in lard. Fortunately, their food options also included vegetables that the slave owners discarded because they did not know how to prepare them, such as collard, turnip, and mustard greens. Within these scraps, slaves received a good portion of their nutritional requirements. Slaves also had the advantage of not having access to the various processed foods their masters may have enjoyed. This is reminiscent of Queen Elizabeth and her royal court's unhealthy eating habits as compared to the poor working class which tended to be healthier.

Revealing the *itis*!

What do all of these foods have in common? They all contribute to what is affectionately known in the African American community as the *itis*. The *itis* is a natural occurrence that happens to individuals after they have over-consumed a meal that is high in refined carbohydrates. Many Americans know that around the middle of November there is a certain Thursday when overindulgence in our favorite foods brings a special bliss. On this glorious day of gluttony, there is a feast of food and a gathering of family and friends. During this time, there are also several parades, football games, and food comas, also known as the *itis*! For some, this eating behavior happens a lot more often than on Thanksgiving. As fun as it may sound, the *itis* is a rather frightening occurrence once you fully understand what is taking place inside your body.

The term *food coma* reveals a certain physiological truth. When we over consume food, especially food high in processed carbohydrates and sugar, our bodies must fully digest the food we just consumed. In the process, your body uses massive amounts of blood to target a full stomach to assist in digestion. When this happens, the effect is very similar to going out in the cold for too long, and your outer limbs start to get numb because your body is recruiting the blood to target your core, therefore leaving your appendages without blood, resulting in numbness. To focus on the digestion process, your body basically shuts down. You, in turn, go into an almost sedative state—i.e., a sleep state. The medical terminology for this is *postprandial somnolence*. (14) This term refers to when a drastic decline in blood pressure occurs after eating.

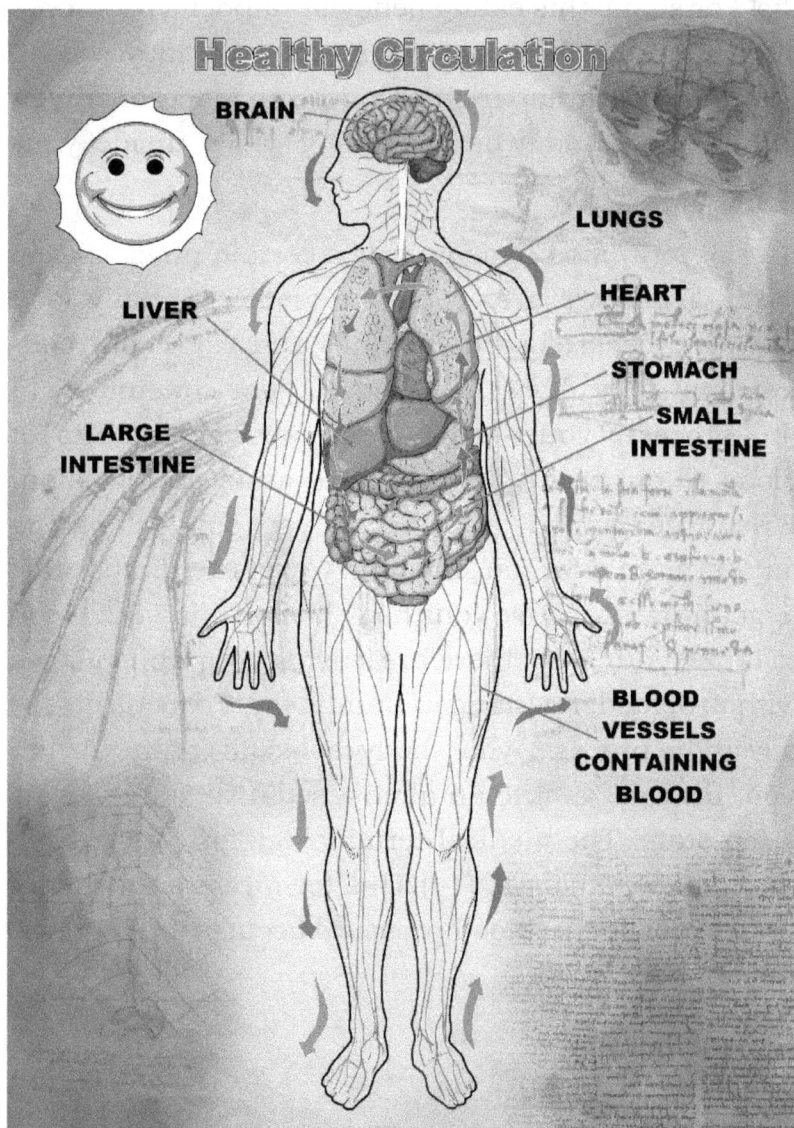

Healthy Circulation

BRAIN
LUNGS
HEART
LIVER
STOMACH
SMALL INTESTINE
LARGE INTESTINE
BLOOD VESSELS CONTAINING BLOOD

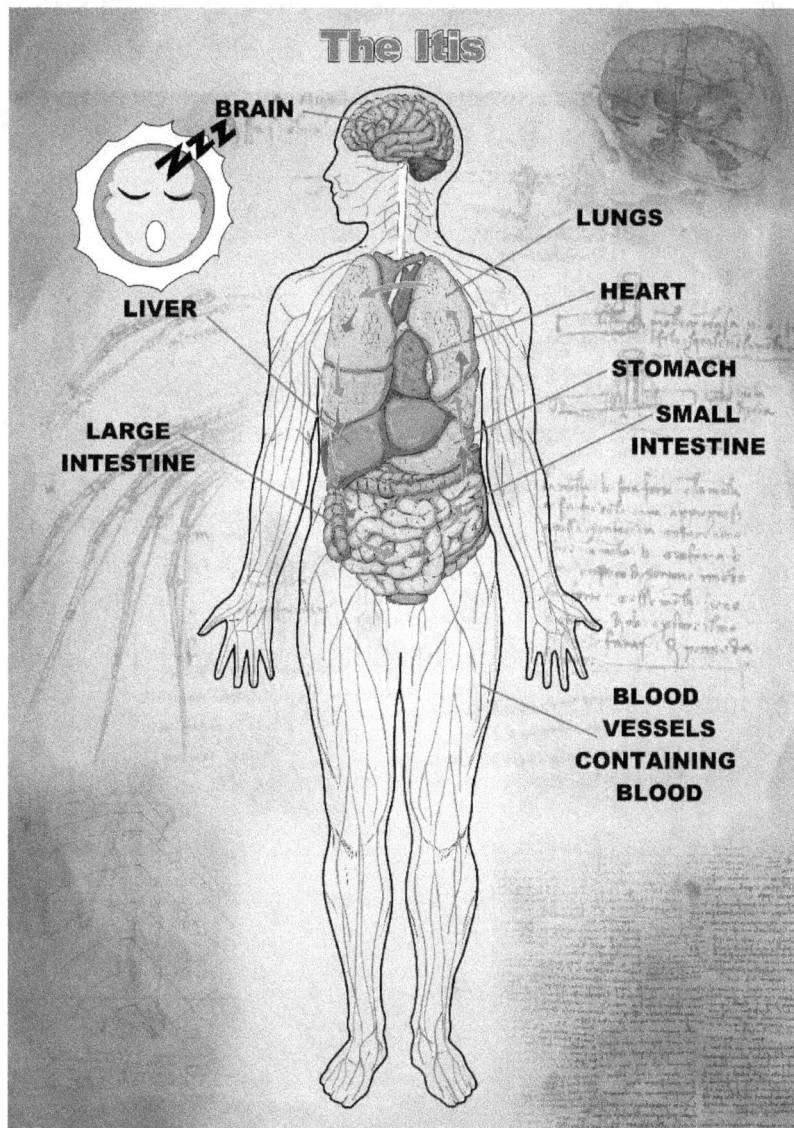

The Itis

BRAIN

ZZZ

LIVER

LUNGS

HEART

LARGE INTESTINE

STOMACH

SMALL INTESTINE

BLOOD VESSELS CONTAINING BLOOD

For as long as I can remember, friends and family would say things like, "You've got that *itis*," or, "I know I am gonna have the *itis*." I never used to think about the origins of this term. But upon further research, I discovered that the origins of the suffix *-itis* are rooted in the Greek, *-ites*. The suffix *-ites* would be combined with another word in Greek, *nosos*, which implied a disease. (15)

In this book, when I refer to *itis*, I am referring to an overindulgence in food that leads to a food coma. Interestingly, overindulgence in processed and sugar-laden foods can manifest as a host of various diseases. This leads to our current state of unhealthy lifestyles that not only plague African Americans and many other cultures but ALL Americans. Unhealthy eating is often a result of socio-economic conditions for many communities and cultures.

CHAPTER 3

WE ARE DRINKING AND EATING OURSELVES TO DEATH!

In Between the Sheets

A few years ago, I was at my old low-carb, low-sugar store, Whoa . . . That's Lo!, and a very interesting customer came through the doors. She was an older, attractive woman who was dressed well, had a great personality, and was totally ecstatic about the store and all the products we carried. As I was helping her peruse products and decipher, based on my experience, what I thought were quality goods, we started talking and she began to tell me about her past. From her appearance, you would not have thought she struggled with alcoholism, and she definitely didn't look like someone who had been strung out on drugs. However, she discussed her addiction struggles with me and her ability to regain control of her life.

At the time, the most surprising thing about our conversation about her struggle with addiction was when she said that sugar was harder for her than to quit drugs or alcohol! She recalled that several times when she was living a sober life, she would wake up at night with a bag of cookies next to her, not remembering how they got there. Her sugar craving was so strong and illustrates her lack of control, even while asleep, to resist sugar! Her story sheds light on the addictive power of sugar. Years ago, I learned that alcoholics aren't chemically dependent on beer, wine, or liquor. Their bodies are addicted to the *conversion* of alcohol into *sugar*. Upon hearing this, I was completely blown away because at this time, I was also researching sugar's addictive nature and how it relates to fungus, which I will discuss later.

In today's modern world, with the advancements in drugs and technology, we seem to forget about the most technologically advanced machine ever created in the history of mankind: our body. We were only blessed with one, and it's a shame that we often treat our "iGadget" with more care! Among some of the most terrifying things happening in our country is the growing number of prediabetics and type 2 diabetics as well as the obesity epidemic, which is seen in both adolescents and adults. It is important to note that once an individual becomes overweight, there is an increased probability of having more health-related issues. With that said, the types of foods these individuals consume kick open the door to a host of potentially fatal diseases.

The following is a list of alarming US statistics that warrant a deeper look at your health as well as the health of your family and close friends:

- 25.8 million children and adults, which is 8.3 percent of the population, have diabetes.
- 18.8 million people have been formally diagnosed with diabetes.
- 7.0 million people are undiagnosed.

- **79 million people in our country are pre-diabetic. (This is almost 25 percent of the US population!)**
- Heart disease is noted on 68 percent of diabetes-related death certificates among people aged sixty-five or older.
- Strokes are noted on 16 percent of diabetes-related death certificates among people aged sixty-five or older.
- The risk for stroke is two to four times higher among people with diabetes.
- In adults twenty or older with self-reported diabetes, 67 percent have blood pressure greater than or equal to 140/90 mmHg or use prescription medications for hypertension.
- Diabetes is the leading cause of new cases of blindness among adults ages twenty to seventy-four.
- Diabetes is the leading cause of kidney failure, accounting for 44 percent of new cases in 2008.
- 48,374 people with end-stage kidney disease also have diabetes.
- 202,290 people with end-stage kidney disease, due to diabetes, are living on chronic dialysis or with a kidney transplant.
- 60–70 percent of people with diabetes have mild to severe forms of nervous system damage.
- More than 60 percent of nontraumatic lower-limb amputations occur in people with diabetes.

- 65,700 nontraumatic lower-limb amputations are performed in people with diabetes.
- $174 *billion* is the total cost associated with diagnosed diabetes in the United States.
- Factoring in the additional costs of undiagnosed diabetes, prediabetes, and gestational diabetes brings the total cost of diabetes in the United States to $218 billion! (1,2,3)

Today, many Americans suffer from diabetes, making it an epidemic. The above statistics provide a real glimpse into the horror of diabetes in the US.

Recently, there has been a major increase in wrongful police killings of unarmed minority citizens in the United States. Technology, largely due to cell phone videos or police officers' body cameras, has increased the public's awareness of these killings. My intention is not to discuss, debate, or critique police killings, as I feel that police officers have one of the most challenging and high-stress-level jobs on the planet, and I couldn't imagine being in their shoes on a daily basis. However, the wrongful killing of any unarmed and defenseless person is unacceptable and, sadly, gets swept up under the rug, with many officers, literally, getting away with murder. It is unnerving.

With that said, I researched data on the number of police-inflicted deaths and compared it with the number of deaths related to diabetes. The statistics are alarming. The amount of legislation and community work needed to combat these tragic police killings is complex; however, the number of deaths resulting from diabetes (being listed on the death certificates of our nation's citizens) is something we can begin to put a stop to now, at this very moment! (4,5)

Historically, this "epidemic" has, sadly, hit the African American and Latino communities hard, and it still plagues these communities today. Diabetes among minorities has become one of the largest health epidemics in the United States. As the minority population grows, so does the number of reports of diabetes and chronic kidney disease. I often think that just as the hip-hop culture in the US was primarily rooted in African American and Latino communities, diabetes was originally "rooted" in these communities too. I often recall my African American friends and family members saying, "You got the sugar (diabetes)?" I make this analogy between the hip-hop culture and diabetes to illustrate how like hip-hop, diabetes has gone mainstream.

Being in the health and fitness industry for over twenty years, I have witnessed how diet and a sedentary lifestyle impact not only one's waistline but also, more importantly, one's life. Diet choices are absolutely contributing to enormous health issues for an existing and growing segment of the US population. New immigrants, who adopt a more Western diet when they settle in the United States, increasingly run their chances for obesity and type 2 diabetes by consuming cheap processed foods. This is a direct correlation between poor food choices and subsequent health issues:

Diabetes is an urgent health problem in the Latino community. Their rates of diabetes are almost double those of non-Latino whites. Getting information to the community about the seriousness of diabetes, its risk factors, and those who may be at risk, and ways to help manage the disease is essential (American Diabetes Association). (6,7)

CHAPTER 4

THE UNHEALTHY
VEGETARIAN

○●○

How Can You Work Here!?

I was working at my family's store, Laurel Health Foods, and saw a gentleman in one of the grocery aisles looking around. I greeted him and asked if there was anything I could help him find. He was looking at the various packages of organic rice and grains we carried at the time. He mentioned a rather peculiar item that I was unfamiliar with. Upon looking at my shelves, we didn't seem to carry it. During our conversation, he was quick to point out that he was a vegetarian and wanted to add this item to his food options. He asked if I was a vegetarian. I politely told him no, "I'm a proud meatatarian!" He looked shocked and then went on to ask me how I could work at this establishment. Now mind you, this gentleman had a huge gut. I began to explain to him that just because you claim to be a vegetarian doesn't mean that you've been knighted by the Health King. I eat organic and grass-fed protein and tons of fresh organic vegetables as well as fruits. I have had various conversations with folks like this, and much of the time these self-proclaimed vegetarian experts are in fact overweight. They might not eat animals, but they are definitely eating something! I understand that this may not pertain to all vegetarians, vegans, or ovo-lacto vegetarians. But in my years of experience, I have come across my fair share of individuals who claim to be vegetarians while looking as unhealthy as someone who lives at McDonald's.

This chapter may ruffle a few people's feathers. My aim is to address a very common misconception that not eating meat means you're automatically healthy. Some people don't consume animal protein due to religious or deep personal beliefs. But simply eliminating meat doesn't make you healthy. If you're not careful, a vegetarian lifestyle can still be unhealthy.

In my opinion, the vegetarian diet tends to be misleading and sounds as if vegetarians are healthier because they don't eat meat. Just because you don't eat meat doesn't mean you're not overeating. Individuals who are clearly overweight or suffer from food related illnesses are most likely consuming foods that are high in sugar and/or foods that convert into sugar quickly due to their high carb count, regardless of it being a vegetarian option.

I am a proud flexitarian and view good-quality protein as a very important building block for optimal health. However, I do enjoy consuming a wide variety of fresh organic vegetables along with various fruits. First, let's look at what defines a true vegetarian, as I've encountered folks who claim to be vegetarian but still eat fish. They are *not* vegetarians, but rather *pescatarians*, which means they eat seafood but no poultry or meat. They often think this title deems them healthy, but if you don't follow a balanced diet, then you are not truly healthy regardless of what you eat. For example, if you eat fish and chips five times a week, then you are not making smart food choices. If you intend to live a lifestyle void of meat and chicken and possibly fish, then I want to shed light on the true meanings of these styles of eating:

1. Vegetarian: The Oxford English Dictionary defines a *vegetarian* as "a person who does not eat meat or fish."

2. Vegan: Veganism is a type of vegetarian diet that excludes meat, eggs, dairy products, and all other animal-derived ingredients. Many vegans also do not eat foods that are processed using animal products. Most vegans also avoid the use of all products tested on animals as well as animal-derived non-food products such as leather, fur, and wool. The term *vegan* refers to either a person who follows this way of eating or to the diet itself. (1)

3. Semi-vegetarians, a.k.a. **FLEXITARIANS**: Semi-vegetarians either limit their intake of certain types of meat or the amount of meat. For example, they might not eat red or white meat, (beef, pork, venison, etc.), but instead, eat fowl and fish. Or they might only eat meat once or twice a week. Someone who only eats fish as a protein source can also be called a *pescatarian*.

4. Ovo-lacto vegetarians: Ovo-lacto vegetarians do not eat any animals, but they do eat eggs and dairy products.

5. Raw/living foodists: Raw or living foodists eat only raw food because enzymes are destroyed by normal cooking processes.

6. Fruitarians: Fruitarians eat only fruit and fruit-like vegetables (e.g., tomatoes, cucumbers), and sometimes seeds and nuts. (2,3,4,5)

As you can see, there are several terms for various food choices. Whether you choose to eat meat or not, I recommend adopting a lifestyle that includes balanced foods that are clean and free from antibiotics, pesticides, hormones, and steroids. I believe there are unhealthy meat options, and I do my best to avoid them. I no longer consume pork as I feel it's a very dirty animal and will literally eat anything given to it. I also steer clear from all fast-food chains because the quality of the food isn't very good. I have had several experiences over the years where I've foolishly given in to my hunger pains and visited a fast-food spot only to have the meal, (if you can even call it that), that within 40 minutes, comes right back up to say hello. Granted that's only happened a few times, but each time it not only reminded me of how poor quality the food is, but also how clean I eat and that my body is not tolerating that type of low-quality food. When you really look at meat as something that is unhealthy, it is not the "meat" per se, but rather the way the animal was raised and then slaughtered. If it is an option, I would always consume food that is less processed, contains fewer artificial ingredients and hormones, and is organically raised free of pesticides.

As human beings, we have been consuming animal protein for thousands of years, and we've definitely been eating meat in America prior to its discovery by Europeans. The following illustrates a brief history of vegetarianism:

- The earliest records of (lacto) vegetarianism come from ancient India and ancient Greece in the sixth century BCE.
- Following the Christianization of the Roman Empire in late antiquity, vegetarianism practically disappeared from Europe.
- During the Renaissance, vegetarianism re-emerged and became more widespread in the nineteenth and twentieth centuries.
- In 1847 the first Vegetarian Society was founded in the United Kingdom. Germany, the Netherlands, and other countries followed.
- In 1908, the International Vegetarian Union, a union of the national societies, was founded.
- During the twentieth century, vegetarianism grew in the Western world because of more nutritional, ethical, and, more recently, environmental, and economic concerns.
- Currently, sixteen million people in the US do not eat *any* animal products.

- Vegetarianism is increasing rapidly in this country. In 2009, 1 percent of the US population was vegetarian. Five years later, 5 percent of the US population is vegetarian. (6,7)

If you choose the vegetarian lifestyle, be mindful of your calorie intake. Make sure your choices are free of sugar and processed carbohydrates. When I was growing up in my family's health food store, there were very few packaged groceries available. I remember meeting people in the store and they would tell me how they eliminated meat from their diets for health reasons. However, I noticed many of them gravitated to foods that were not as healthy as they thought. Many of the food choices mentioned were instant meals, cereals, desserts, snacks such as chips, fruit juices (even though natural, they still contain a lot of sugar), and sodas. Today, there are enough products and companies available to allow for a large chain such as Whole Foods to exist. Some twenty, thirty, or even forty years ago, there would not have been enough merchandise to fill the shelves or support an entity as large as Whole Foods.

With the increase in processed food options that now make eating organic and/or vegetarian easier than ever, we need to peel back the layers of the real culprit behind an ever-expanding waistline and a potentially unhealthy diet. If it were simple to become healthy, then everyone buying organic and vegetarian foods would be at a healthier weight. But when I shop at a local health food store, I don't see this happening. Sure, the overall quality of products is much cleaner in the customers cart, but you'd think there would be leaner waistlines on people shopping in the grocery aisles. I tell people all the time that you can buy organic, frosted, sprouted grain vegan flakes or good ol' Tony the Tiger Frosted Flakes, and the only difference is that one is made with cleaner and "healthier" ingredients, but they are both still loaded with sugar and processed carbohydrates! It's like the difference between smoking environmentally friendly, organic, and free trade cigarettes or smoking yucky cigarettes. You're still smoking cigarettes!

There are a ton of products on the market that are now riding the organic label bandwagon. If you don't know what ingredients to look for, you're just going to spin your wheels. Later in the book, I will explain how, once and for all, you can stop waistline expansion with a formula I like to call Zillion-Dollar Math. In the next chapter, I will explain what organic truly is and will illustrate the differences between organic and non-organic foods, many of which you may already be aware of.

CHAPTER 5

WHAT DOES ORGANIC REALLY MEAN?

○●○

According to Organic.org, (and you can't get more organic sounding than *that*), *organic farming* is "agriculture that does not use chemicals, genetic modification, or irradiation, using only natural products. The term *organic farming* was first printed in the 1940 publication *Look to the Land* by Lord Northbourne. Organic farming is not just a technique, but a philosophy as well." (1)

Eating organic can be very expensive. If you have a compromised immune system, you should do everything in your power to buy organic. If you don't have a compromised immune system, don't worry if you can't afford to eat everything organic. It's better to eat a non-organic salad than a basket of cheese fries. Grocery shopping for a family of four can be challenging, but when you add in the organic food items, the grocery bill can add up very quickly. Below are a few tips and strategies that I use whenever I am on the hunt for groceries.

Buying Organic on a Budget

- Most large-scale supermarkets these days have their own privately labeled line of organic packaged foods, from frozen peas to organic turkey bacon, and even organic canned corn. You just have to keep an eye out for the products because the labels might not be familiar. The products will be in the same general area as the major brands. Even Whole Foods offers an entire line of their own privately labeled groceries and these options can be considerably less expensive than the name-brand companies.

- In the DC, Maryland, and Virginia area, we have been experiencing a boom in discount grocery stores like Aldi and Lidl. The shopping format may be a little different from what we Americans are used to; however, the savings are incredible! Not only are the products discounted, but they also carry full product lines of organic packaged foods like fresh produce, organic meats, eggs, and dairy products.

- You may not think about organic groceries when you shop at TJ Maxx, Marshalls, or even Burlington Coat Factory, but you'd be amazed at the selection of organic products that they carry. Now, you won't shop there for organic milk or eggs, but I typically purchase very high-end olive oils, snacks, coffee, and even protein powders from these retailers. The only downside is that they may not consistently carry the same brand, but to me, organic olive oil is organic olive oil!

- Lastly, nothing makes me more excited than seeing organic chicken that has that special "clearance" sticker on the front! The chicken has been drastically marked down due to the expiration date swiftly approaching, but for me, that's like hitting the organic lottery! The chicken is fine, but the supermarket needs to try to sell it at a discounted rate before the expiration date. I've scooped up several packages of chicken that would normally cost $7-10.00 for $3.00! If I am not using it before the expiration date, I simply throw it in the freezer until I need it.

There is a group called the Environmental Working Group (EWG) that publishes a list each year of produce with the top 12 highest pesticide residues and produce and the top 12 with the least amount of pesticide residues and produce. This list is a great resource and something you should consider when shopping. Below is the list EWG published in 2018:

12 Most Contaminated Foods (2)

1. Peaches
2. Apples
3. Sweet bell peppers
4. Celery
5. Nectarines
6. Strawberries
7. Cherries
8. Pears
9. Grapes (imported)
10. Spinach
11. Lettuce
12. Potatoes

12 Least Contaminated Foods

1. Onions
2. Avocado
3. Sweet corn (Frozen)
4. Pineapples
5. Mango
6. Asparagus
7. Sweet peas (Frozen)
8. Kiwi fruit
9. Bananas
10. Cabbage
11. Broccoli
12. Papaya

In my opinion, we don't have to get fanatical about whether all of our foods are organic. The main point is to become more conscious of what organic is and how it can benefit your body. When you are shopping and looking at produce and meat selections, for example, look for sales on items you may otherwise purchase as non-organic, or try a new food that is on sale and experiment with a new recipe! Personally, I've noticed a difference in taste between organic and non-organic foods. After a while, you will see yourself becoming conscious about the quality of the foods you consume.

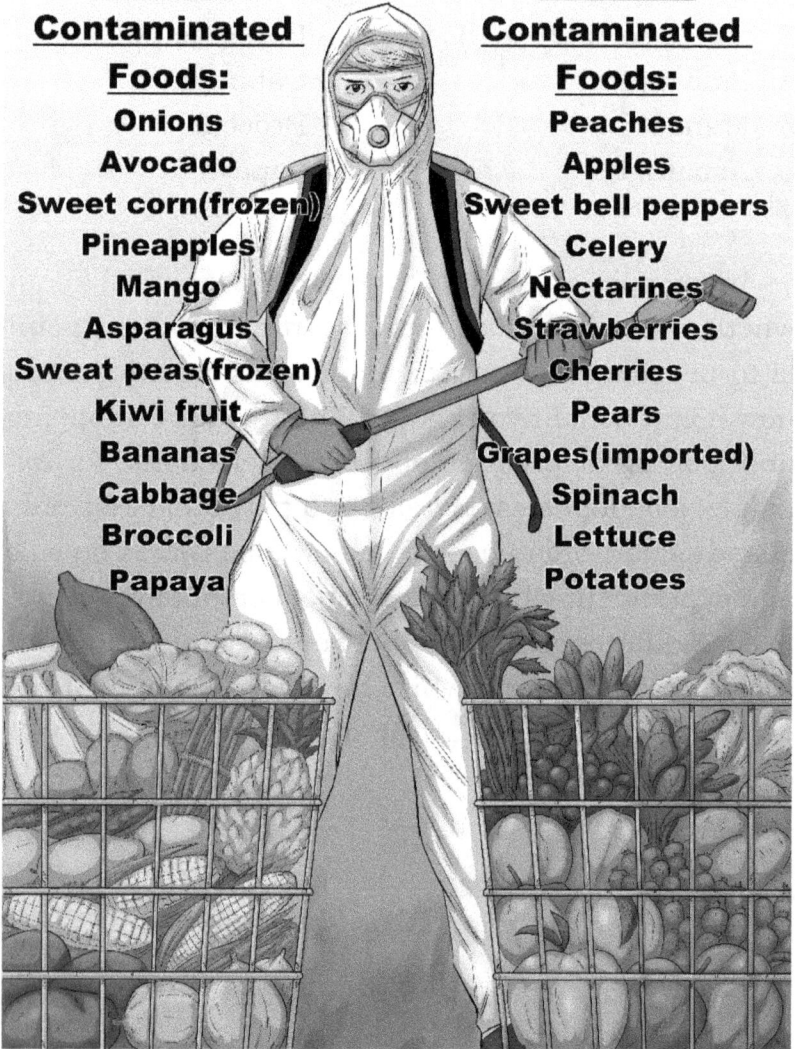

12 Least-Contaminated Foods:

Onions
Avocado
Sweet corn(frozen)
Pineapples
Mango
Asparagus
Sweat peas(frozen)
Kiwi fruit
Bananas
Cabbage
Broccoli
Papaya

12 Most-Contaminated Foods:

Peaches
Apples
Sweet bell peppers
Celery
Nectarines
Strawberries
Cherries
Pears
Grapes(imported)
Spinach
Lettuce
Potatoes

CHAPTER 6

ZILLION-DOLLAR MATH

○●○

Zillion-Dollar Math!

Ladies and gentlemen, the following mathematical computation will *change your entire life*. When the Dr. Atkins products first started hitting the shelves around 2000, I couldn't help but notice that there was a weird phrase on the back of the products. It was located near the nutritional label and generally at the bottom right underneath or next to it. This phrase was two words—*net carbs*—and it was always followed by a number. Before we illustrate the computation, let's look at a few keywords on the nutritional label you must pay attention to:

Dietary fiber

Carbohydrate

Sugar alcohol

Serving Size

The term *net carbs* refers to the following mathematical calculation:

Subtract the total dietary fiber from the total carbohydrates and then subtract any sugar alcohols (if listed), which will equal the net carbs.

The net carb number is the number of carbohydrates that will convert into sugar and spike blood sugar levels. Since fiber and sugar alcohols have a minimal impact on blood sugar levels, they can be subtracted.

My Zillion-Dollar Math Formula should primarily be implemented for processed foods. As I noted earlier, processed foods include chips, sodas, juices, candy bars, granola bars, bread, and pasta, or essentially, anything that is manufactured and put into a package. For non-processed or foods that are in their natural state and have not been altered by man or machine, this rule does not warrant the same amount of attention. Non-processed foods (fruits, vegetables, nuts, seeds) typically have a lower impact on one's blood sugar levels.

AT-HOME EXPERIMENT

Let's review this process by reading different packaged food labels that you have at your disposal. You probably have bread, (or some other packaged food), in your kitchen. Do the following:

1. Locate the nutritional label on the packaging.
2. Find the total carbs listed (in grams).
3. Find the total fiber listed (in grams).
4. Subtract the total fiber from the total carbs.
5. This number is the net carbs.

Formula Breakdown:

Total Carbs - Total Fiber = Net Carbs. The net carbs are what impact your blood sugar levels.

When I did this experiment, I looked at the nutritional labels of Pepperidge Farm Light Bread and Nature's Own Wheat Bread. Here is what I discovered:

ZILLION DOLLAR MATH

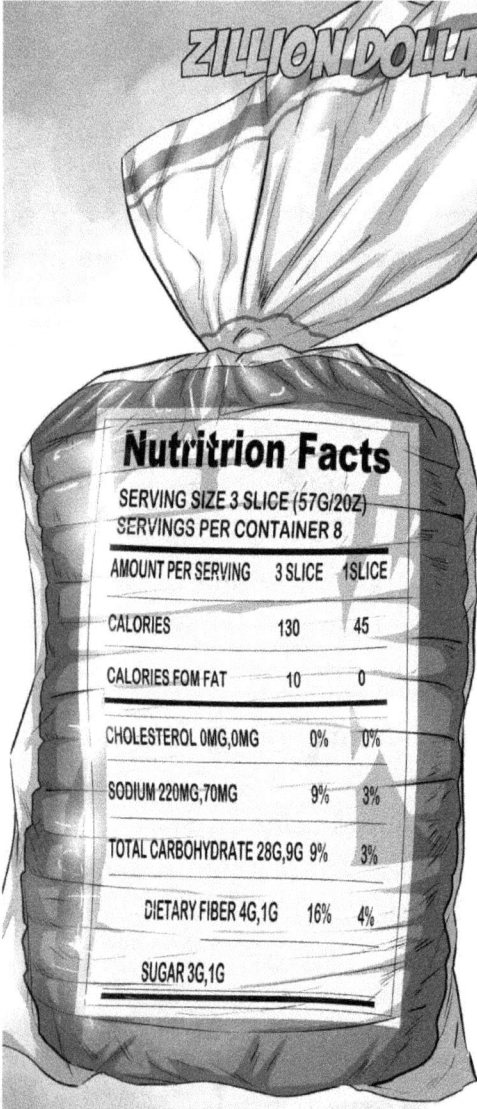

Nutritrion Facts

SERVING SIZE 3 SLICE (57G/2OZ)
SERVINGS PER CONTAINER 8

AMOUNT PER SERVING	3 SLICE	1 SLICE
CALORIES	130	45
CALORIES FOM FAT	10	0
CHOLESTEROL 0MG,0MG	0%	0%
SODIUM 220MG,70MG	9%	3%
TOTAL CARBOHYDRATE 28G,9G	9%	3%
DIETARY FIBER 4G,1G	16%	4%
SUGAR 3G,1G		

**PEPPERIGE FARM
LIGHT BREAD**

**TOTAL CARBS: 28G
TOTAL FIBER : 4G
NET CARBS:
24G PER 3 SLICE
OR 8G PER SLICE!!!!**

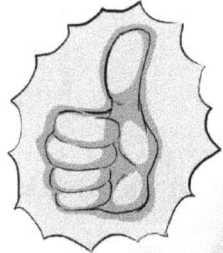

ZILLION DOLLAR MATH

NATURE'S OWN WHEAT BREAD

TOTAL CARBS: **18G**

TOTAL FIBER :   **2G**

NET CARBS: 16G FOR 1 SLICE OF BREAD!!!!

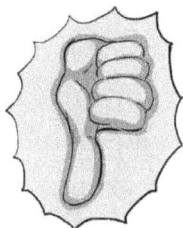

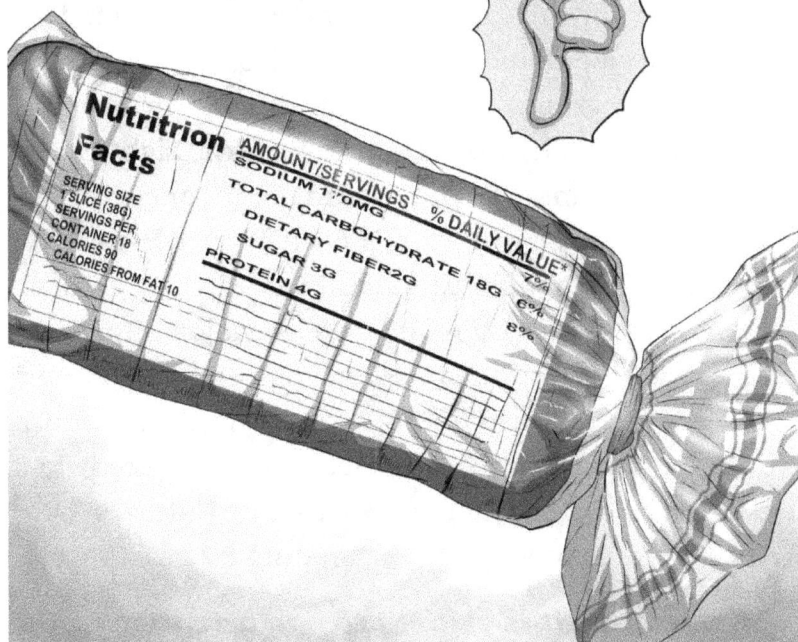

The *X* grams of net carbs are going to convert into sugar once they are consumed. Obviously, the preferred choice in this scenario is Pepperidge Farm Light Bread, with only 8 grams per slice compared to Nature's Own's 16 grams per slice. I personally try to stick to a net carb number of 10-15 grams or lower. If I need to decide between two different types of bread or any packaged food, I use the Zillion-Dollar Math Formula and choose the lesser of the two evils after doing this calculation.

The total carbs minus dietary fiber is the number to monitor in terms of spiking blood sugar levels. The other thing to be mindful of with packaged food is the serving size. If you applied the same math for what we previously calculated for the sliced bread, we would consume 24 grams of carbohydrates in one serving, which is *three* slices of Pepperidge Farm Light Bread versus 16 grams of carbohydrates in one serving, which is *one* slice of Nature's Own Wheat Bread. We can apply this simple calculation to making a sandwich and see how this can have a major impact on your choices. If you made a delicious sandwich using the Pepperidge Farm bread, your net carb count would be 16 grams for the bread on your sandwich. However, a sandwich made with the Nature's Own Wheat Bread would have a whopping 32 grams!

Remember, it is critical to pay attention to the serving size on the label of ALL packaged foods!

I use this formula when comparing processed foods. If the food is manufactured or processed, the net carb number is typically higher. I don't pay as much attention to net carbs when it comes to fruit and vegetables. However, sometimes I may choose blueberries over a pineapple. Why? Because pineapples naturally have a higher sugar content than blueberries, and it is wise to be mindful of the sugar intake from fruits and certain vegetables.

As the low-carb diet craze grew, so did the various products that made their way to the shelves. *Net carbs*, *impact carbs*, and various other terms landed on packaged foods hoping to inform consumers of the potential spike in their blood sugar levels. When you consume carbohydrates, you have an increase in blood sugar levels. Carbohydrates that are not burned as energy are stored as fat. Therefore, eliminating carbs will help you lose weight because your body burns stored fat for energy. What makes my Zillion-Dollar Math Formula so powerful isn't the math itself, but the ability to apply this simple formula to anything and everything manufactured on the planet for human consumption! Heck, I've even looked at it for my dog's treats.

In America, we are more fascinated with calories and fat numbers on the back of the food labels than the numbers that make up the net carbs of a product. If an item has a low net carb count, then the other numbers such as calories are low as well. Paying attention to these numbers, applying the Zillion-Dollar Math Formula, and making different food choices could simply be the difference between fitting into your pants or putting those pants in the "someday" pile. This could also be the difference between keeping all your appendages or having a toe surgically removed because of type 2 diabetes. The risk of serious health-related issues such as obesity, type 2 diabetes, hypertension, and high blood pressure decrease when smarter, healthier food choices are implemented.

After looking at countless labels over the years, 10 grams of net carbs is a good number to base your decision on for packaged food choices. When you choose a packaged food, do the calculation to find the number of net carbs, and if a food is more than 10 grams per serving, you should consider an alternative. If it is 10 grams or less, sit back and enjoy! But if you don't pay attention to the serving size on the label, you could easily consume over 30 grams of net carbs and not even realize it!

When most people start to pay attention to food labels, they often come to a scary and surprising realization that they have been consuming high amounts of processed carbohydrates, sugars, calories in relation to serving sizes, and in turn, potentially sabotaging their health. If you are one of these people, don't worry, so was I. Once I removed the blinders, I became empowered and in control of what I was consuming. Whether I was in a grocery store, eating out at a restaurant with friends, or in a random convenience store, I started to see food from an entirely different perspective. The Zillion-Dollar Math Formula illustrates the importance of paying attention to the nutritional content of processed foods. It allows you to make better food choices quickly and effectively, which leads to a healthier lifestyle.

CHAPTER 7

THERE'S FUNGUS AMONG US!

○●○

Let's Talk About Fungus

Fungal toxins in the food we eat represent the number one worry we face as a human race.
—Simon Shane, LSU Press, 1991 (1)

The primary food source for fungus is sugar, which is why we often crave something sweet! Our bodies are not actually telling us that we need chocolate, soda, bread, or crackers. Instead, the fungus is releasing mycotoxins to stimulate you to feed the fungus, this is why we have a sweet tooth. We don't crave fiber or calcium or any other important nutrients in this way, but unfortunately, we often crave donuts or cake or some other type of food that contains sugar. (2)

Another interesting thing to note is that alcoholics are not chemically dependent on wine, beer, or liquor. In actuality, their bodies are chemically dependent on the alcohol converting into sugar. When someone wins the battle against alcohol addiction, it may be common that they suddenly have a "sweet tooth." (4) The fungus has just found a different form of delivery to get its fix of sugar. Perhaps your drink of choice was a rum and Coke, and now you crave Skittles! My intent is not to make light of the serious nature of alcohol addiction, but to bring awareness to the powerful nature of food addiction, especially as it pertains to sugar and the fungi that feed off of this food.

Most women are aware of *Candida albicans*. *C. albicans* is a diploid fungus that grows both as yeast and filamentous cells and is a causal agent of opportunistic oral and genital infections in humans. *C. albicans* lives and is detected in the gastrointestinal tract and mouth in 40–60 percent of healthy adults." (3) There are approximately two hundred strains of fungus and yet, in America, we only screen and test for about four of them. Have no fear, I am not going to turn this into a science lesson, but I want you to be aware of what we are up against.

By now you may be wondering, "what's up with all this fungus talk?" The focus of this discussion is to bring awareness to addictive behavior that occurs through excessive sugar consumption from processed carbs and sugar-laden foods, which leads to an increased amount of fungus in the body. Here is a rather unpleasant but accurate thought, my mom always said, "when you take your final breath and your spirit finally leaves your body, and they seal the casket and you're buried to rest, the worms and parasites don't enter in through the sealed casket. In reality, they were inside you all along." From the time we are born until the time we die, we carry a multitude of organisms in our bodies, known as fungi. The fungus feeds off of poor diet choices. The goal is to decrease fungi in the body by restricting its preferred food choices, namely sugar. By informing you of what is truly causing cravings, we can finally attack and destroy the food source of our fungal culprit, sugar, which as I have repeated throughout this book, is one of the most addictive drugs on the planet!

The best way to kill off fungus in the body is by eliminating its primary food source. By dialing in on what we are consuming and drinking, we can drastically restrict the food source of the fungi. But in doing this, it is important to note that they won't go without a fight!

A Herxheimer reaction occurs when a fungus dies. This can happen by restricting the food source for fungus, which is sugar and processed foods. By eliminating the food source, we kill the fungus. A Herxheimer reaction occurs when large quantities of toxins are released into the body as bacteria (typically spirochetes). (5) A Herxheimer reaction reveals itself in symptoms related to the dying fungus. The dead fungus is released into the bloodstream, and you experience withdrawal symptoms such as fever, chills, headache, myalgia (muscle pain), and exacerbation of skin lesions. When you feel better or normal, the fungus has left the body through the bloodstream.

The same can be true for candida death when toxins from the dying candida are released. Typically, the death of these bacteria and the associated release of endotoxins occur faster than the body can remove the toxins. The intensity of the reaction reflects the intensity of the inflammation present. (6) The intensity of the withdrawal or of the Herxheimer reaction illustrates how large of a fungal problem the individual may have.

If you ever have taken an antibiotic, more than likely you have ingested a strong fungus, because that is what antibiotics are made of. *Biotic* is Latin for "life," and *anti* is defined as "against or opposed to." When taking an antibiotic, essentially, you destroy good bacteria.

You will never totally rid yourself of all fungus. Think of the Chinese philosophy of yin and yang and its symbolism of balance. As this pertains to taking antibiotics, once you finish a regimen, it is crucial to ingest good, healthy bacteria called probiotics, pro means "for", and biotic means "life". During the course of the antibiotic, you kill most bacteria in your body. You must find balance.

CHAPTER 8

HOW TO START LIVING A HEALTHY LIFESTYLE

◐●◐

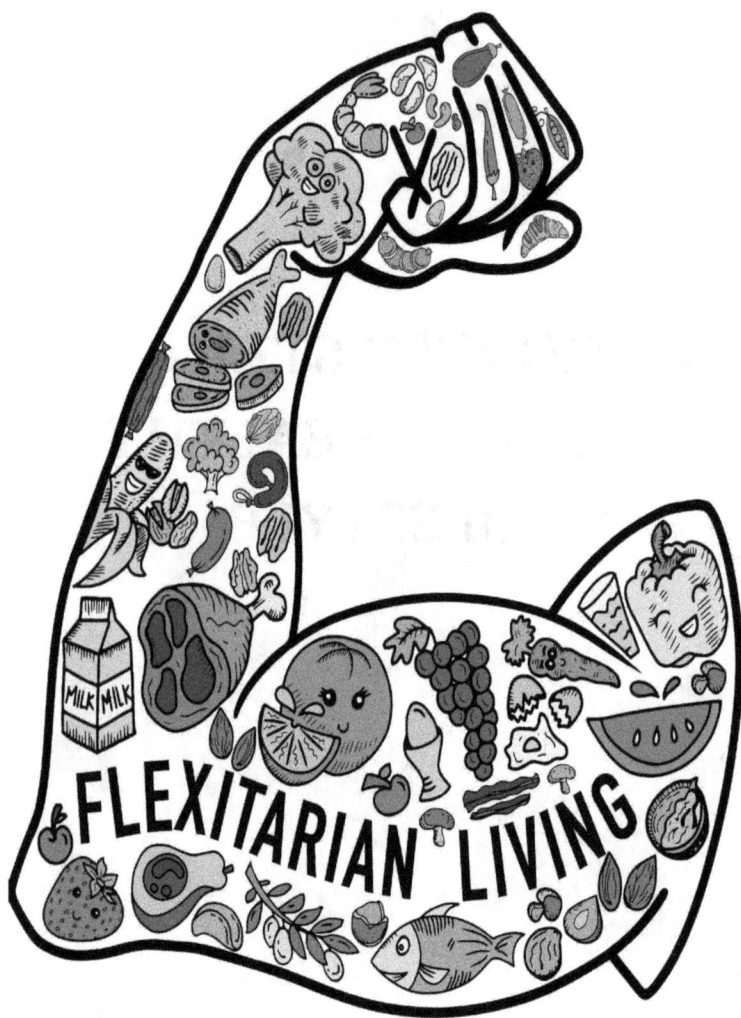

FLEXITARIAN LIVING

Roughly 95 percent of people that have diabetes in this country suffer from type 2 diabetes, while only 5 percent suffer from type 1 diabetes. According to the American Diabetes Association, type 2 diabetes is explained below:

Diabetes is a problem with your body that causes blood glucose (sugar) levels to rise higher than normal. This is also called hyperglycemia. Type 2 diabetes is the most common form of diabetes. If you have type 2 diabetes, your body does not use insulin properly. This is called insulin resistance. At first, your pancreas makes extra insulin to make up for it. But over time, it isn't able to keep up and can't make enough insulin to keep your blood glucose at normal levels. (1)

With type 2 diabetes, genetics and lifestyle are the two factors that contribute to the development of this disease, with an unhealthy lifestyle leading the charge.

According to the American Diabetes Association, type 1 diabetes is explained below:

Type 1 diabetes is usually diagnosed in children and young adults and was previously known as juvenile diabetes. Only 5 percent of people with diabetes have this form of the disease. In type 1 diabetes, the body does not produce insulin. The body breaks down the sugars and starches you eat into a simple sugar called glucose, which it uses for energy. Insulin is a hormone that the body needs to get glucose from the bloodstream into the cells of the body. (2)

You wouldn't believe the number of people I talk to who accept diabetes as a natural part of their lives. They explain that diabetes runs in their family. In most situations, I am talking to people who suffer from or have family members that suffer from type 2 diabetes. It's as if they've already given in to the fact that they have a special diabetes family gene and there's nothing they can do about it. Proactive behavior toward your health and wellness can drastically reverse type 2 diabetes as well as a host of other health ailments. These illnesses include high blood pressure, high cholesterol, and obesity.

Small steps can be taken to reduce the likelihood of developing type 2 diabetes. I will explain this by using something I call flexitarian living. The term flexitarian is not new. This term was introduced in 2003 as being the most useful word, according to the American Dialect Society. (3) As previously defined in chapter 4, a flexitarian consumes a plant-based diet and eats meat occasionally. I perceive a flexitarian lifestyle as being more than just food consumption. Flexitarian living can be applied to all facets of one's life with a focus on flexibility. I've witnessed many people becoming too rigid in their behavior toward new diets and/or fitness programs. This can result in stress both mentally and physically. Being flexible with your exercise program and what you're going to eat for lunch today as well as not having to take supplements every day allows you to stop self-sabotaging and start living a truly healthy lifestyle. This is where the concept I call the Four Pillars of Health comes into play.

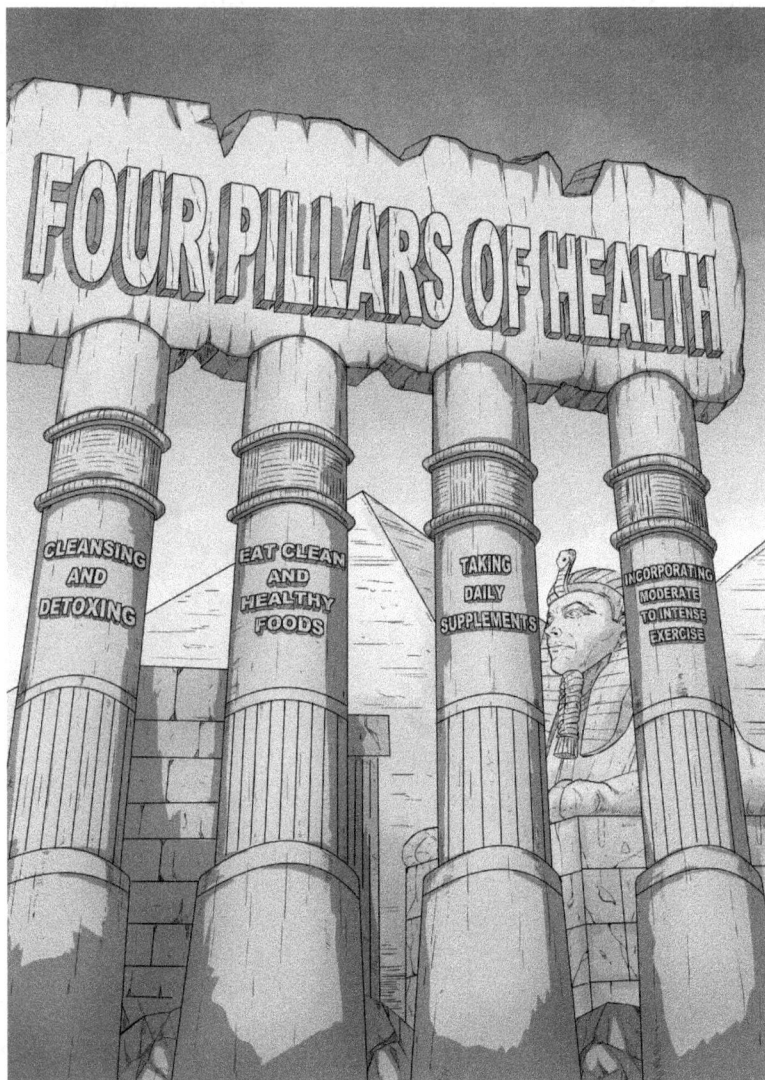

Incorporating the Four Pillars of Health into your way of life is a major component in helping to deter the development of diabetes and other diseases.

Flexitarian Living Revealed

Thus far, I've shared the detrimental role sugar has played throughout history and the impact it has on our current society. In this chapter, I will explain how to begin living a flexitarian lifestyle. Each of the Four Pillars of Health can help assist with sustaining vitality and overall good health while alleviating stress.

Pillar 1: Cleansing and Detoxing

Cleansing is a critical component of flexitarian living. Start with a clean slate. Getting rid of all the junk and toxins in your body is essential for good health and longevity. In reality, these are two separate processes.

Focusing on a good cleanse at least once a year helps rid your body of food that collects in the ridges of the large and small intestines and helps cleanse many of the vital organs. This results in better absorption of the nutrient-rich healthy foods you eat. You'll also have better absorption of the supplements you take.

Most people look at cleansing as something they may get around to doing one day; then there are those that have been sold on various "diets" that are built around cleansing for quick results and dropping un- wanted pounds. If you are overweight and looking to lose weight, keep in mind that you didn't gain all your weight overnight, so you're not going to lose the weight overnight either! Contrary to popular belief, a good cleanse will not send you running to the bath- room. Consider this analogy: Every three thousand miles or so you schedule an oil change. If we drive our automobiles without ever taking the time to change our oil, the car will eventually start to smoke and grind to a halt. Luckily, you can replace an automo- bile; you cannot as easily replace your body.

Here are some common things to keep in mind about cleansing:

- **Drinking plenty of water is essential during cleansing/detoxing the body.** If you do not consume sufficient amounts of water while consuming high amounts of fiber, the exact op- posite can happen and instead of flushing out, you can become extremely constipated.
- A good cleanse is *not* a laxative and will not send you running to the bathroom.
- Flexitarian living restricts food sources that fungi and other parasites feed on, which also helps you cleanse.
- During my personal cleanse period, I tend to restrict the amount of animal protein I

consume and lean more toward a pescatarian diet. This is also one of the benefits of being "flexible" with your diet, hence a flexitarian lifestyle!

- You can experience a sense of "withdrawal" and an increased desire for sweets when you restrict sugary, processed foods.
- Depending on how poor your current diet is, you may experience nausea, chills, and flu-like symptoms.
- Once your body eliminates toxins through the cleansing process, you will begin to feel better.
- I don't promote a specific cleanse or detox because there are so many on the market today.
- Try to cleanse for a period of 7-10 days.

Pillar 2: Eating Clean and Healthy Foods

Although Dr. Robert Atkins popularized the low-carb movement that I am a big proponent of, he missed a golden opportunity to emphasize that the real culprits are *sugar* and *refined carbohydrates*. We can give him credit for helping us become more educated about good fats and good cholesterol, but there are still some people who are unaware of this fact. In America, we have become conditioned to think that all fat and cholesterol are bad. My second pillar of flexitarian living, Eating Clean and Healthy Foods, exposes people to the world of good fat, good cholesterol, and healthy carbohydrates that are all critical to over-all health, weight loss, and maintenance.

You're Gonna be Mad at Me!

A few summers ago, I had the opportunity to meet with a group of local middle school children who were learning about healthy eating. I took it upon myself to show them how to decode the mysterious and deceptive nutritional labels. They were very surprised to see that what they thought was one serving turned out to be one and a half or in some cases, two servings for many foods. Many of the kids had various tall cans of sweet tea and a few had a soda can. When they started to turn the cans around to look at the labels, many couldn't believe what they saw! For 1 serving, the carbohydrate/sugar count was easily around 20 grams. What floored them was when they realized that a tall can of tea was 3 servings, which made consuming 1 can a total of 60 grams of sugar!

Taking notice of serving size is a huge piece of the healthy lifestyle puzzle. It is key to educate kids at an early age about nutrition and health. During my visits to schools, I always love seeing young people involved in taking action and showing an eagerness to learn how to be healthy. This will, hopefully, lead to decreased numbers of childhood and adolescent obesity.

That school year, I was invited back and was presented with a Certificate of Appreciation. After I said a few words about diabetes and obesity, I could see that many of the parents should have been the ones attending my lecture that took place during the summer. Once everything was over, the principal looked over at me with great hesitation and announced that there were cake and refreshments, a.k.a. soda, in the back of the room.

Many parents approached me and thanked me for that talk and for teaching their kids about nutritional labels. Some shared that they had diabetes in their families. One lady in particular, talked to me about her husband's type 2 diabetic condition. I could see the true concern on her face as she shared the challenges she experienced trying to get her husband to take better care of himself. Not long into the conversation, a moderately overweight man (her husband) approached us. He stood behind her and looked at me and grinned saying, "You're going to be mad at me!" Once he came into full view, I could see that he was holding a plate of cake. To make matters worse he had two big slices of cake with super heavy frosting on his plate, which was much more than an individual serving. As he stood there playfully joking about me being mad at him, I began to explain to him that I wasn't the one eating the cake! In fact, I could have afforded to eat both pieces if I chose to, but someone that is clearly overweight and has been clinically diagnosed as a type 2 diabetic should not. This man is a classic example of a person addicted to sugar.

Clean and Healthy Food Pyramid

During the height of the low carb boom, an explosion of books on this subject started to flood the bookstores. I had the opportunity of inviting Fred Pescatore, M.D., the author of <u>The Hamptons Diet</u>, to Whoa...That's Lo! LLC for a book signing. During this time, there was a lot of talk about how the FDA Food Pyramid was all wrong and some experts even talked about flipping it upside down. What I loved about <u>The Hamptons Diet</u> was that Dr. Pescatore re-arranged the various food groups into their own respective pyramids! I have always found this fascinating, and his pyramids also help determine healthy food choices. All you need to do is stick to the base of each pyramid and you're eating healthy foods. As soon as you start to consume foods higher up on the pyramid, the health benefits start to decline. I included 4 pyramids and did some modifications to them for you to use as a guide when you are choosing what to eat. To me, these 4 pyramids create the foundation of food options for adopting a flexitarian lifestyle regardless of whether you lean toward eating like a Vegetarian or a Meatatarian. Simply eat the base of any of the pyramids and you're instantly consuming a healthy selection of foods. I also highly recommend Dr. Pescatore's book because he goes into detail about the various healthy fats and highlights the health benefits of consuming those fats.

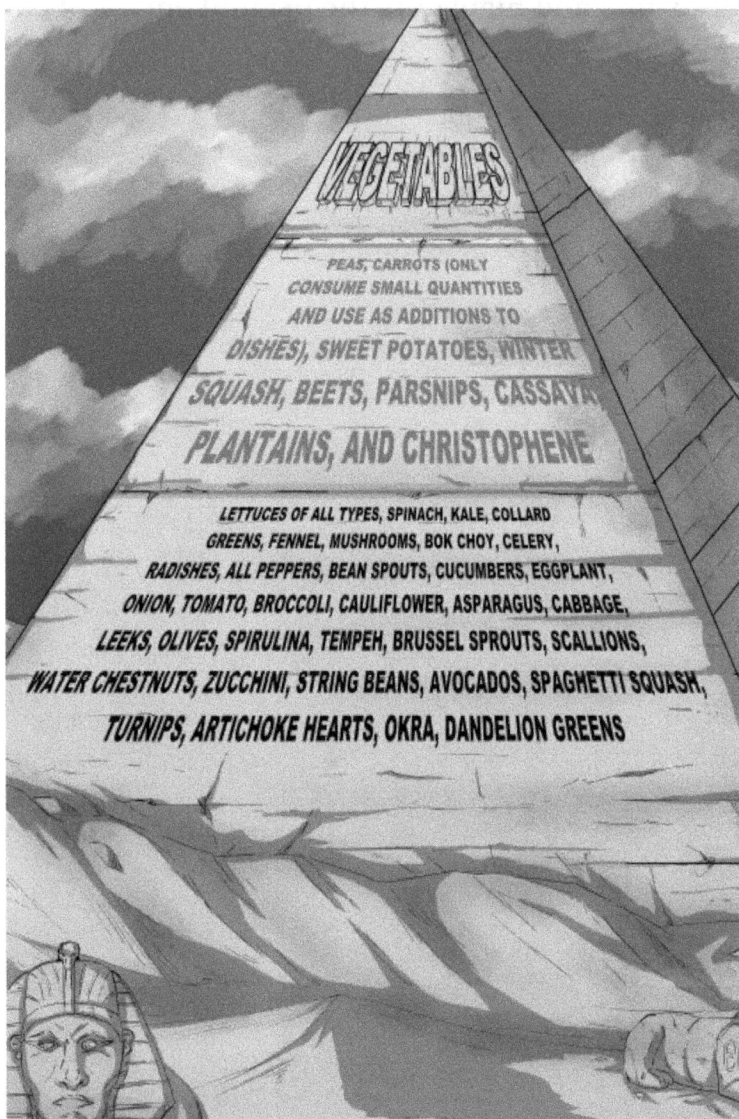

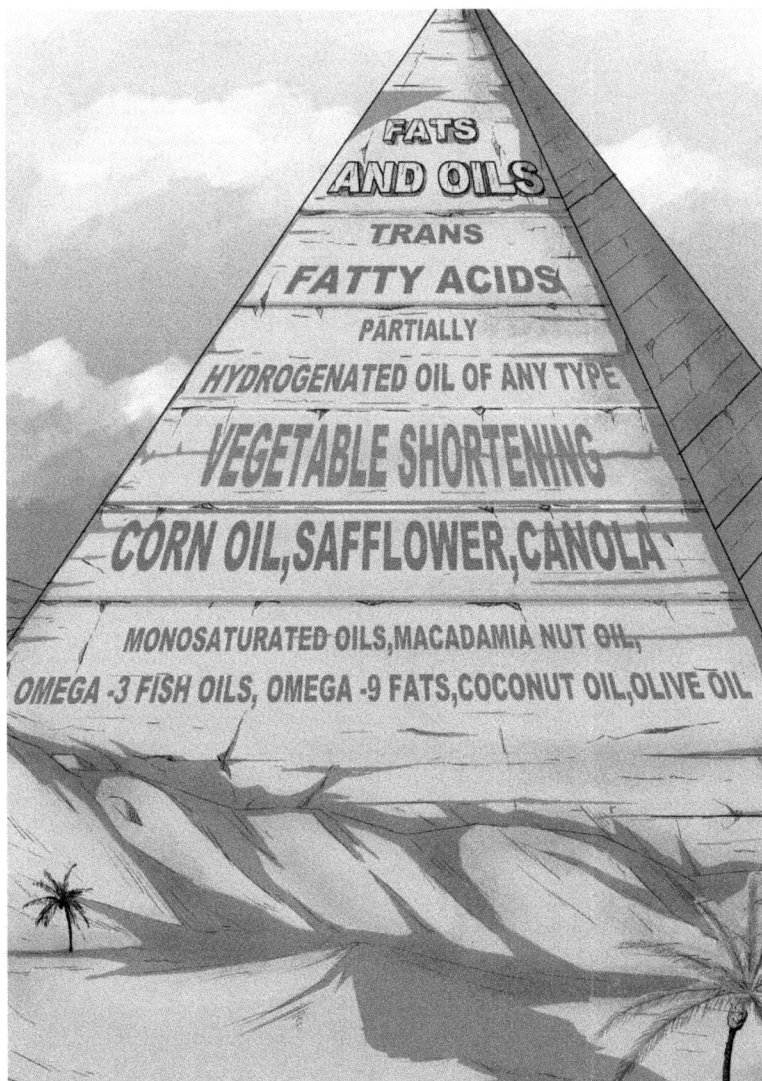

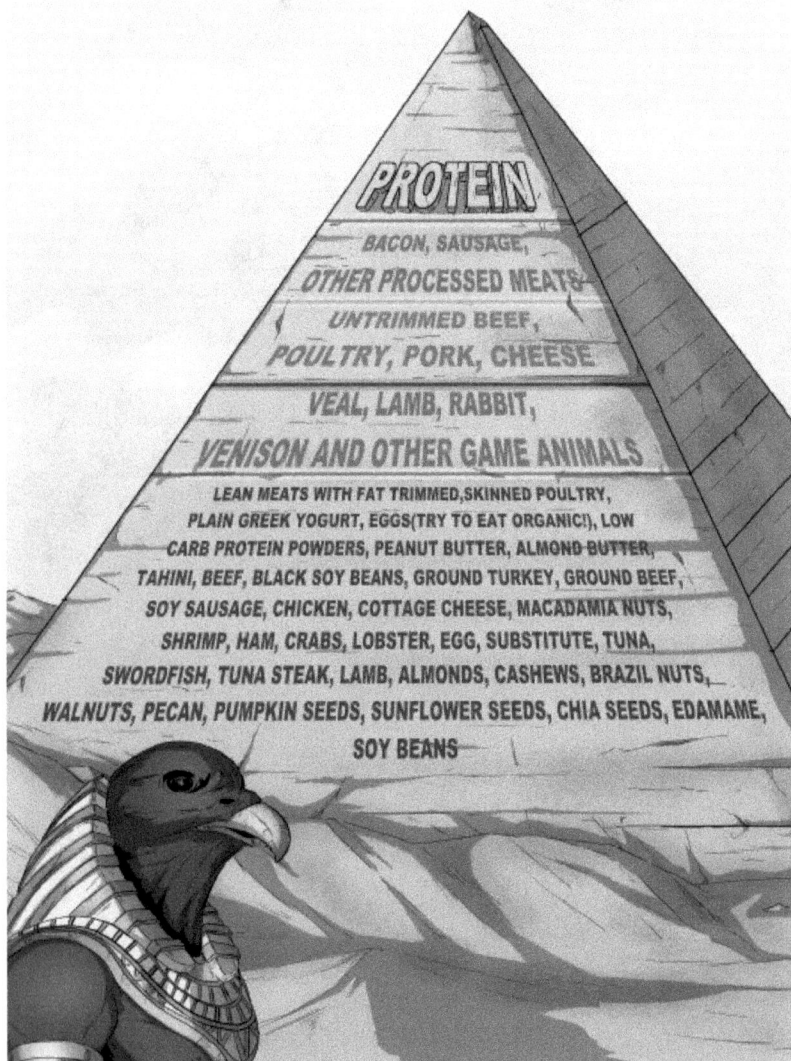

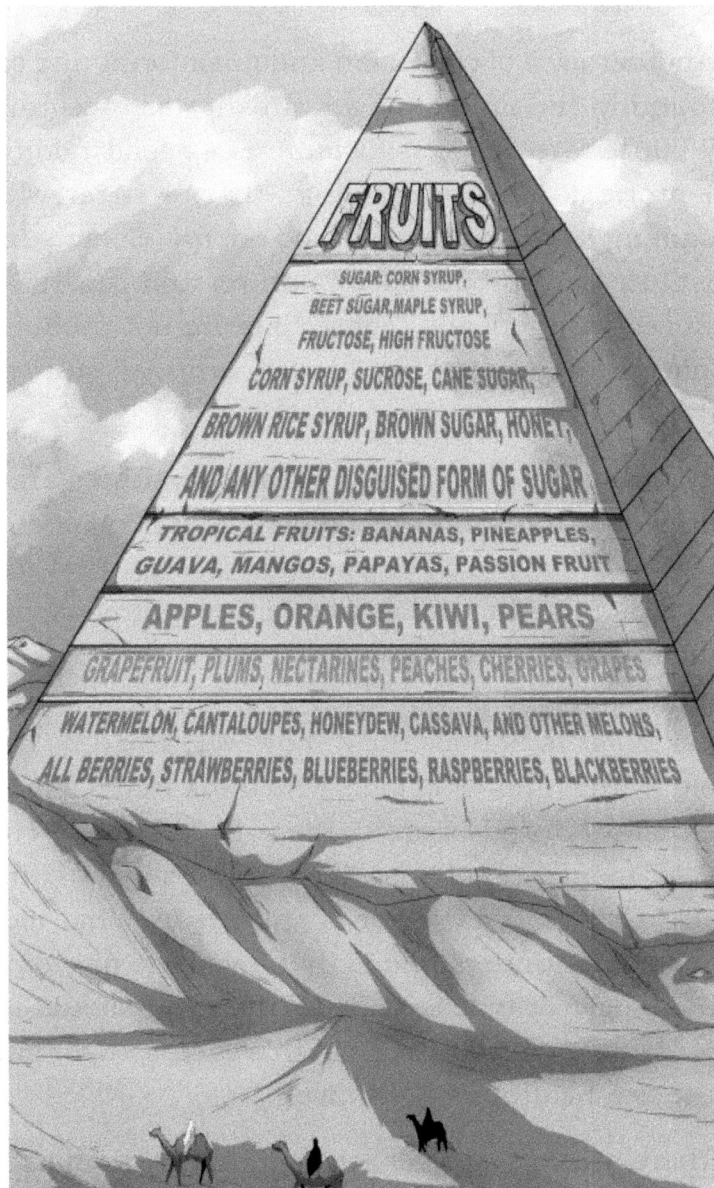

(4,5,6)

The Real Deal on Sugar Substitutes!

Another area of confusion and misinformation can be found in the land of sugar substitutes. According to Wikipedia, a *sugar substitute* is "a food additive that provides a sweet taste like that of sugar while containing significantly less food energy. Some sugar substitutes are produced by nature, and others are produced synthetically. Those that are not produced by nature are, in general, called *artificial sweeteners*.(7)

You may have heard that sugar substitutes aren't healthy and that some are dangerous. When I opened my first low-carb food store, countless natural food sales reps talked to me about the unhealthy aspects of sugar substitutes. However, sugar substitutes are healthier in some cases. Many people are aware that actual sugar is bad for them; however, you'd be surprised by the number of folks who think that if a product is natural and organic, then it's healthier. That sort of mentality is just plain old "sugar-coating sugar." Organic, raw sugar is still sugar. What most people do not understand is that if you are pre- or an actual type 1 or type 2 diabetic, then you should not be consuming *any* sugar. So in this case, a sugar substitute *is* a healthier alternative.

There are better, safer, cleaner, and more natural sugar substitutes on the market, such as stevia and agave, to name a few. The problem is that if you're dining out or at a convenience store, the likelihood of you having access to organic stevia-sweetened alternatives is very remote. This is where I choose to pick my battles. If I had to drink a soda, tea, or juice, I would opt for the sugar-free and/or diet alternative. But ideally, I would not consume sodas, or any beverage sweetened with sugar or artificial sugar substitutes. Some might look at consuming artificial sweeteners as unhealthy and dangerous, but I honestly think that all the obesity and health problems occurring at alarming rates around the globe aren't from the overconsumption of synthetic sugar substitutes. They are from the overconsumption of sugar. It took me quite a long time to get to the point of consuming minimal to no soda or sweetened beverages.

Sugar Substitute Tips

- Stevia is a plant and is naturally sweet. The problem with various stevia products is that they can have a slightly bitter aftertaste. The other thing to keep in mind is that a little goes a long way. Someone who uses 2 packs of sugar may only need half of a pack of stevia. There is a company, NuNaturals, that in my opinion, makes the best stevia powder and liquid. No aftertaste! I love their liquid and will literally only need to use a few drops in my coffee. This also helps the bottle last a long time.

- Agave is also a plant and can be found mainly in a liquid form. Again, a little goes a long way so you'll need to experiment with the amount that will suit your needs. Agave can have a gas/laxative effect on some people who have sensitive stomachs so watch yourself!
- Maltitol and Lactitol are both sugar alcohols and are probably the most common sweeteners that you'll find in a lot of the sugar-free candies on shelves across the country. I can't stress this enough but these products can definitely have a gas/laxative effect on your body if you eat a lot! If we ever meet, ask me about the time when I first got in a shipment of sugar-free brownies for the low-carb section of my family's health food store. I didn't have a clue as to what maltitol was then, but I definitely knew after inhaling two brownies!
- Experiment! There are a lot of sugar-free substitutes on the market these days. Everyone's taste buds and preferences are different so what works for some may not work for all. Go out and try a few various products and find what works best for you.
- Lastly, if you are beginning your sugar-free substitute journey, your taste buds will have to go through a major adjustment! I can't remember the last time that I drank a regular sugar-loaded cola, but I can assure you as soon as it would hit my mouth, I would probably be very

sick due to the excessive sweetness and the strange sensation that my taste buds would experience. Over time, what you may think tastes horrible in the beginning won't have that same feeling the more you get used to a new taste.

On the market today, there is a mix of totally organic and all-natural sugar substitutes as well as common and not-so-common synthetics. Eventually, the goal is to eliminate all unhealthy sugars and/or unnatural substitutes in favor of agave or stevia, and to begin to lower your intake of sweeteners overall. Ultimately, the decision of what you consume is up to you, but if you start to eliminate sugar from your diet proactively, you are winning, so keep up the good work!

Pillar 3: Taking Daily Supplements (Boosting Immunity and Vitality)

During my many years working within the natural foods industry, I have seen numerous companies market an unbelievable number of vitamins, minerals, and herbs. The quality of the products offered is as varied as cars, and depending on the manufacturer, you may be "driving" a Kia or a Mercedes Benz. With my expertise, I have created a list of supplements that I recommend. So even if you are taking supplements that are on the lower end of the quality spectrum, you should include the following:

Green food supplements

- It's almost impossible to consume the same amount of raw greens as you can get in a scoop or capsule.
- There are a lot of great tasting options on the market today.
- You can add it to your smoothie. My favorite is to drink it on an empty stomach in the morning.
- These have a super high antioxidant level! *Anti* means *against*, while *oxidant* means *breaking down*. Think of antioxidants as superfoods helping fight your body from "rusting" or breaking down.
- It's great for everyone! From kids to grandparents, there are options for everyBODY.

Probiotics

- As I mentioned earlier in my book, Pro=*for*, biotic=*life*, so when you translate the word, it literally, means *for life*!
- Probiotics put healthy bacteria into our gut, (many people have unbalanced guts).
- Anytime you take an antibiotic, it kills all the bacteria in your stomach/body. It doesn't know what's good or bad. Remember: *Anti* (*against*) *Biotic* (*life*)! So, it's extremely critical to make sure that you're putting the good bacteria

(probiotics) back into your body ESPECIALLY if you have finished taking a round of antibiotics!

- Probiotics are great for everyone! From kids to grandparents, there are options for every-BODY.

Fish and flaxseed oil (e.g., Essential Fatty Acids or EFA'S)

- Just like the greens, the amount of salmon one would have to consume to achieve what a teaspoon of fish oil would be a whole lotta fish!
- If you're vegetarian or vegan, then a good EFA would be your go-to since they tend to be flaxseed and borage, but just check the label to be sure of what you are purchasing.
- EFA products have come a long way! There are a lot of great-tasting liquids or soft gels, depending on your preference.
- EFA's have healthy heart and cholesterol benefits. They are high in HDL (High-Density Lipids or as I like to think about it HAPPY or Good Fat), and not the LDL (Low-Density Lipids or as I like to think of that as SAD or Bad Fat)
- They are great for everyone! From kids to grandparents, there are options for every-BODY.

Magnesium

- This is a very hard-to-consume mineral and is not found in high amounts of daily foods.
- The benefits from magnesium include restful sleep and reduced muscle soreness, and bowel regularity. Magnesium has many health benefits.
- Your body absorbs magnesium during rest so it's good to take it prior to bed.
- Capsules are great but I do enjoy a product called CALM which is a powder that I mix with hot water at night. It is especially nice to drink during the winter months because it's nice to sip before I doze off to sleep.
- Great for everyone! From kids to grandparents, there are options for everyBODY.

These four supplements are very important to maintain a healthy lifestyle. Certain individuals may have to take a vitamin or herb that may address a specific condition, whether it is high blood pressure or diabetes. However, these four supplements provide you with a solid platform where you can launch your healthy supplement program. These four supplements should become part of your routine and the basis of your supplement program. You can begin this program at a young age. I give my children these supplements daily, and in doing this, I am teaching them to understand the importance of this pillar and how it pertains to living a healthy lifestyle.

Pillar 4: Incorporating Moderate to Intense Exercise (Spending Energy Creates Energy)

The definition of moderate to intense exercise depends on the individual. The main emphasis here is that exercise is important, but it's a small piece of a larger puzzle.

By simply changing overall eating habits and incorporating a good selection of supplements, you are going to start to win the battle! If you incorporate exercise, you can really intensify the results that you will soon achieve!

My personal experience with exercise and fitness has been a lifelong journey and I still enjoy pulling myself out of my comfort zone and trying new things. At the end of the day, the most important thing to do is to move more. When you rest, you rust!

The most important thing to do is to move more. Remember, exercise can be anything from parking your car further away, taking the steps instead of using the elevator, or taking a kickboxing class. Below are recommendations to consider:

- Find a gym or training facility that is convenient.
- Make sure the atmosphere or culture is something you want to be part of.
- Do not set unrealistic goals with your training program.

- Periodically set physical training goals, i.e., increase a lift by X pounds in six months or run a mile in X minutes.
- Remember, slow and steady wins the race.
- Become passionate about your fitness.

One important thing to remember, it's just a workout! Flexitarian living embraces the healthy lifestyle journey and understands that within this journey, you may not have perfect training days 365 days a year. You should have fun and enjoy the experience, or else you may eventually stop. Look at your fitness as physically taking your body to the next level. The next level can be walking a mile, running a marathon, or competing in your first triathlon race. Just get up and get moving!

Big John

A few years ago, I had an older gentleman inquire about my new gym and training program, CrossFit Laurel. At first, I was a little skeptical that he would actually take me up on a free intro session and if he did show up, that he would even join. So the day finally came, and John showed up ready to give this whole CrossFit thing a try. He showed up wearing the latest cutting-edge workout apparel that consisted of sneakers, blue jeans, and a long-sleeve plaid thermal shirt! Yeah, you just read that correctly! Well, needless to say, he quickly became a regular and consistently attended my 4:00 p.m. class three to four times a week for almost a year. Time went by and John really started to get stronger. At one point, he was able to deadlift over two hundred pounds. For a guy in his sixties, that was one hell of an accomplishment, and he truly loved the training.

Then one random afternoon I got a call from his assistant letting me know that something serious had happened to John. I could hear the fear in her voice, and she informed me that John was in the hospital. She went on to say that the only people he'd given permission to see him were his girlfriend, his assistant, my brother, and me. She told me that they'd administered his last rights and I needed to come ASAP! I got off the phone and my heart sank. I started to think of the last time I had trained him, and I wondered if I had pushed this guy to his deathbed. I literally dropped what I was doing and headed to Baltimore, MD, where the hospital was located. I really can't explain my emotions upon my arrival, as I had no idea what I was about to walk into. When I stepped into the room, he was asleep and hooked up to more machines than I can even explain. Once he woke up, I could immediately tell that he was in pain but was super excited to see me. He began to explain to me what was going on.

He essentially had a stroke, and once he was admitted to the hospital, they realized one of his femur bones had cracked. Several weeks prior, I had John on a special training device we use called a GHD (glute hamstring developer), and that supposedly "caused" the fracture. I say "caused" because he went on to explain that he had a very serious cancer of the blood that he was totally unaware of. John had no clue his femur had been broken, which was because cancer had softened his bones. He went on to tell me that muscle had built up around his legs making them stronger. This was the reason he didn't fall over once the fracture occurred. The doctors also informed him that his heart being so strong from his training was another reason he was still alive.

If the stroke had happened to anyone else with the same disease and at his age, they would have died from the stroke. Needless to say, he couldn't thank me enough! I really couldn't believe what I was hearing, and as happy and excited as we both were, John was nowhere near being out of the clear. The doctors still didn't think he was going to make it out of the hospital. I came back the next day, and when I walked into his room, it was hard to fight back the tears that began swelling. John was knocked out again, but on the wall directly across from his bed, he had our CrossFit Laurel T-shirts taped up on the wall along with an old photo of him running in a marathon. John woke up and happily greeted me, saying with a big, eager grin, "Hey, man! Well, I made it another night. These damn doctors can't believe it!"

Time went on, and Big John continued to amaze doctors and various medical experts. He continued personal training sessions with me on and off for the next few years. It truly saddens me to write this, but due to the growing intensity of his cancer and because it had weakened his bones, it became more challenging for John to move around. One day, John had a fatal fall and sadly passed away. Big John was a close friend, a mentor, and a true supporter, believer, and member of the CrossFit Laurel family.

I put this story in here to hammer home that fitness isn't just about being half-dressed and taking selfies to post to Instagram. Sure, you can use whatever you want as a tool for motivation. The reasons can go on and on—from wanting to look better naked to being able to carry a wounded person out of a hostile situation. I like to think of our bodies as well-oiled and fine-tuned machines. This machine, handcrafted by the greatest builder in the universe, begins to rust if rarely operated! I encourage everyone to find some sort of physical activity that keeps you moving, regardless of age. The younger you can start, the better! And folks out there with children, you have even more reason to be active. This not only will have a profound and powerful effect on you, but more importantly, on your children and their children for generations to come. For Big John, taking action for his physical health and well-being saved him and added a few precious years to his life.

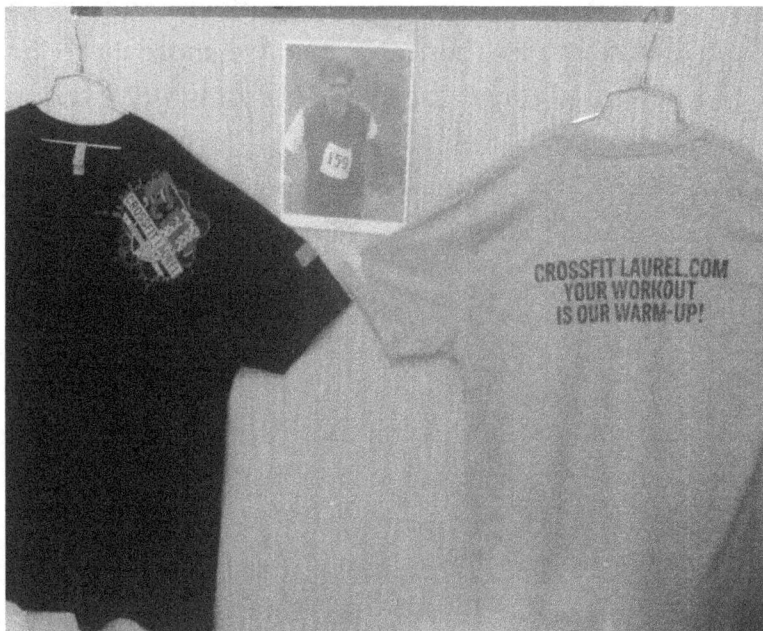

CHAPTER 9

HEALTH AND VITALITY CAN BE YOURS

○●○

Laila's School Assignment

One afternoon I was picking up my little princess from kindergarten, and when I arrived, I could see she was super excited to, of course, see her DaDa, but there was something else she was pumped up about. She started to tell me about a healthy eating worksheet that her class had to complete and as soon as we got into the car, she pulled it out of her backpack with a big smile, beaming from ear to ear.

She began to explain what the assignment was all about and how she answered 100 percent of the answers correctly. The assignment was to draw lines from various types of foods that were healthy and wanted to eat, to an empty plate. For breakfast, she chose fruit, eggs, and bacon and didn't choose cereal, pancakes, donuts, or the cinnamon bun. For lunch, she selected sliced apples, carrots, and peas. She didn't choose the burger, fries, pudding, chocolate chip cookie, or chicken nuggets. She did make it a point to explain that she was considering the nuggets, but because they had breading on them, she left them off but did recognize the protein benefits. For dinner, she selected steak, broccoli, and corn. She didn't select the biscuits, pie, pizza, mashed potatoes, or rice. I immediately started to praise her on a job well done and told her that I was extremely proud of her. At that time, she was only five years old and had a solid understanding of what healthy whole foods were, compared to unhealthy processed foods!

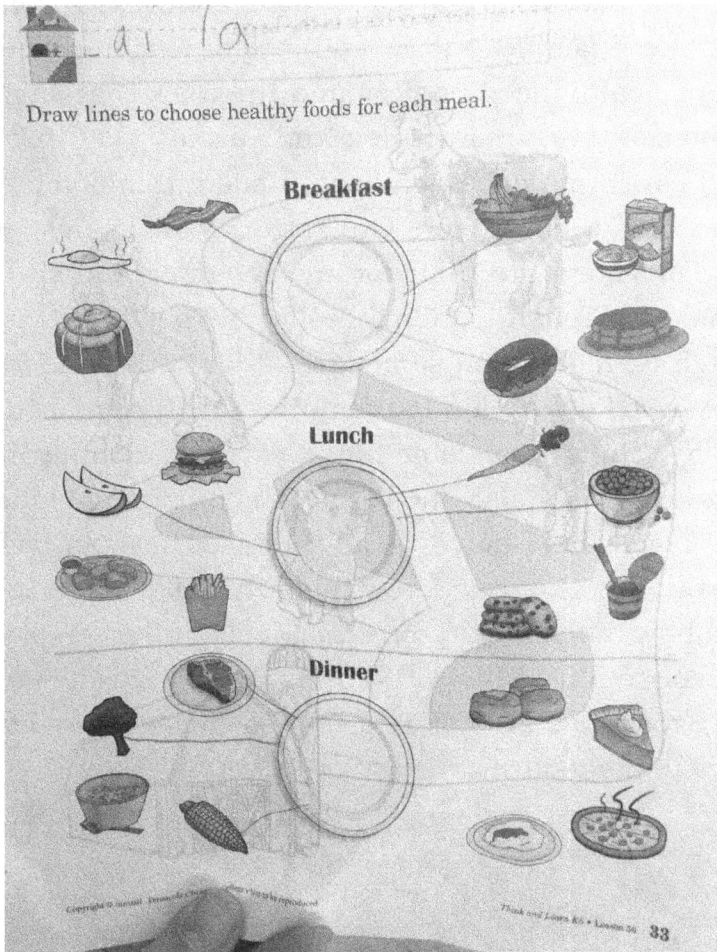

Draw lines to choose healthy foods for each meal.

I wanted to include this story for a few reasons. First, I love my daughter and told her I was going to put that story in my book, and what proud dad wouldn't want to brag about his amazing child? Second, I want to bring to your attention the fact that this is how you can finally end the unhealthy family syndrome that plagues so many of us today. I always knew that when I started to have children, I would lead by example and would begin teaching them about healthy food choices and the roles that sugar, protein, water, fresh fruits, and veggies play in our food consumption. I don't try to make things too extreme for them either. On Saturday mornings, it's kind of a standard thing for my kids to have a bowl of Cinnamon Toast Crunch cereal while they sit down to watch cartoons, and sometimes, I join in on the fun. However, I do explain to them that this type of food is really a "treat" and something we don't consume on a regular basis. I also show them the nutritional labels and teach them how to read them so they can begin to start to understand how the nutritional labels look and how much sugar, for example, is in the cereal we are consuming. This sort of routine serves as a learning experience as well as a time for me and my little ones to hang out.

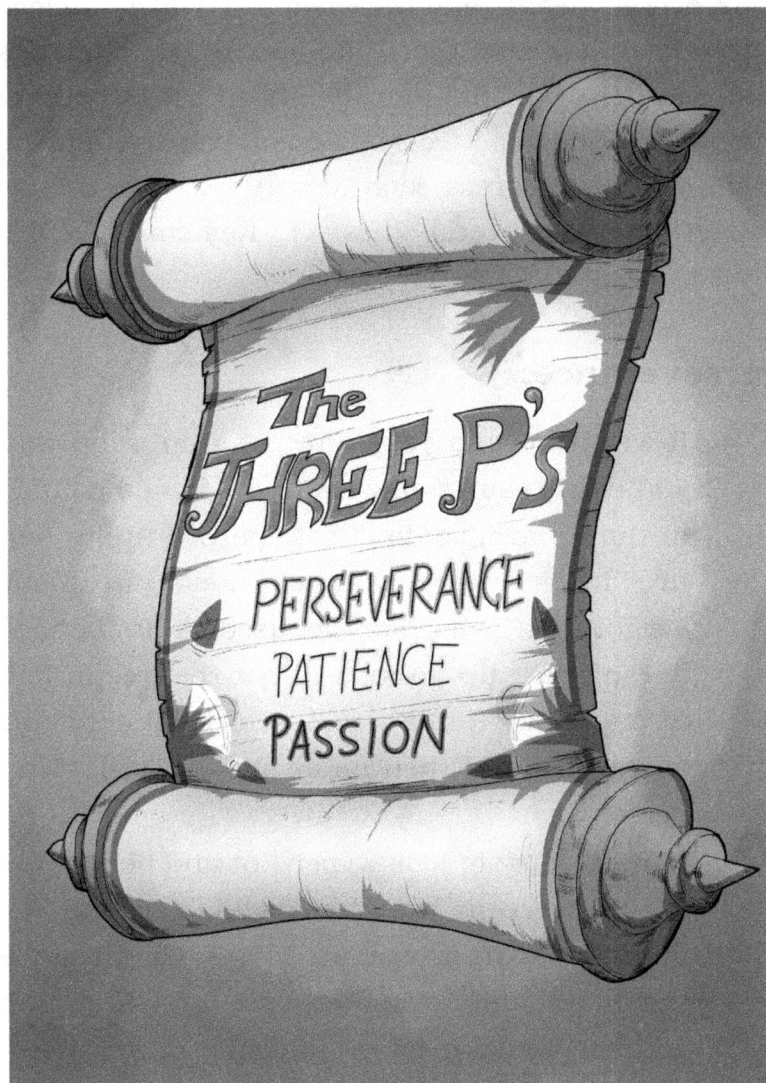

As you begin to take more positive action toward your overall health and well-being, I'd like to close with some basic tips that I like to call the Three P's that can help with the journey ahead. At the end of the day, no one is perfect, but if you can try to make some positive progress each day, it will have a huge impact on your overall lifestyle. Remember, Little Hinges Swing BIG Doors!

Perseverance:

- If weight loss is your aim, keep in mind that you didn't gain X amount of unwanted pounds in thirty days, so don't set yourself up for failure by stressing yourself over unrealistic weight loss goals. Stay focused! A lumberjack doesn't pick up an ax and cut the tree in half in one blow. He or she has to keep chopping away at it, and then he or she can yell, "Timber!"

- If it was easy to look super-hot and be in great shape, everyone would be walking around like that. Any man or woman who has a physique that you admire, whether it's a random person you see walking by or Beyoncé in her latest video, trust me, they work their butts off to look like that! Now, Beyoncé may have personal chefs and trainers at her disposal, but the average person at the gym does not. Either way, they are both, to some degree, dialed into what they choose to consume as well as the intensity and frequency of the physical activity they do.

- Watch out for saboteurs! As excited as you might be about hitting the gym and eating healthier, not everyone is as excited for you, and some folks may even knowingly, or unknowingly, try to take you off your path! Changing your eating habits and physical activity can rub folks the wrong way. Trust me, I've seen it in my personal life as well as with clients I've trained. People will be quick to try to knock your newfound path of health and wellness, so sometimes, as the great Jay-Z once said, "You let your stuff bubble quietly . . . and then you BLOW!"

- If you happen to "fall off" your newfound routine, guess what, it's OK! The health fairy isn't going to appear magically and smack you in the mouth for eating that slice of cake at your company social event! It doesn't mean the game is over and you go back to your old, poor eating habits either. This is where flexitarian living comes into play, not stiff and rigid living! What you will notice is that when you really start to make changes in your eating and fitness, when you do have that slice of cake, you will begin to feel the negative effects of the excessive sugar and carbs, and you may find yourself cutting the serving down. The other thing is that you become more cognizant of your actions because you know you're going to the gym later, and you don't want that piece of cake to sabotage the fitness goals you are working so hard to achieve.

Patience:

- Sit back, relax, and fall in love with the journey ahead. Some days/weeks may be better and seem easier than others, but start to look forward to the overall new path you are forging with your health and wellness. I often witness people who have a negative attitude toward their new health and fitness goals. If you're already sounding negative and you've only put in a few days of effort, more than likely, you'll be right back to your old ways in no time. The great pyramids in Egypt weren't built overnight, so your new health and wellness routine won't just magically happen in a weekend. Be patient and start to enjoy the overall process of becoming a healthier you!
- "LITTLE HINGES SWING BIG DOORS!" Small things like cutting back soda consumption to one a day versus five a day over the course of just one month, can have a huge impact on your health. Or eating a side salad instead of french fries over the course of a month, and

then three months, and then a year can result in your waistline shrinking and your health improving in a major way!

- This one is a major game changer toward your physical goals: set various benchmarks and give yourself around three months to hunt them down steadily and methodically! Like a pack of wild coyotes on the scent of a wounded elk in the wild, you want to hunt that target down slowly and steadily! You may want to be able to run 400 m (one lap around a track) at a good pace but, right now, you are only able to power walk this distance. Then, in a few weeks, you can jog about half the 400 m and before you know it, two months have passed and you're able to jog the entire 400 m. By the end of that third month, you've found your stride and can run 400 m at a good pace. The goal here is to use various physical benchmarks instead of just looking at a scale every morning! This gives you something to go after. To add fuel to the fire, write down your various 400 m times per training session so you can track progress and stay motivated. You can always reference this data and truly track the progress you are making!

Passion:

- Love yourself right now, right where you are regardless of your health and fitness! You just finished reading *The Itis Revealed* by Curtis Price! Get fired up!!! The Almighty Creator only made one of you! Get fired up about this new journey of becoming a healthier you! You only have one body so cherish it and be blessed that you can breathe in the air around you and look up at the sky above you! Enjoy each day you are here and make the best of it!

- Get excited about the new healthier you that you are becoming! See yourself finishing that 5K you entered and acknowledge how accomplished you are going to feel after you catch your breath. Start to envision the new healthier you. Your doctor may even tell you that your lab work has improved and you don't need to be on medication anymore!

- Start to have fun in the kitchen or while eating out and try a new healthy vegetarian dish, for example, if you've never done so before. Get passionate and excited about food options. Research quick and easy recipes, start experimenting with a few meals a week and see how you can start to incorporate cauliflower rice into your meals instead of regular rice. If a dish doesn't work out, it's OK! You tried something new and that's what this journey is all about. If you don't pull yourself out of your comfort zone from time to time, you'll never discover new and healthier alternatives that can be major game changers for your new healthy lifestyle.

- If your gym or physical fitness regime is boring and has you dreading another session, then CHANGE IT! Once again, pull yourself out of your comfort zone and shake things up. If you've never done a spin class at your gym, then go ahead and give one a try! If you have never tried a CrossFit gym because you think it's too crazy and you can't do it because of something a friend or co-worker said, then go see for yourself and try a free class! You never know, you may end up falling in love with it. The point here is to be passionate about your new commitment to living a healthier lifestyle; challenge yourself regardless of what it is. From time to time, we can find ourselves in a rut. By pulling ourselves out of our comfort zone, we can shake our bodies up and kick-start things. Just remember, BE PASSIONATE AND HAVE FUN!!!

With these three P's, I hope you are more inspired as you chart a course toward your journey of healthy living. I can't thank you enough for your support. I wish you nothing but the best and hope you have an awesome time on your journey toward living a healthier life!

CONCLUSION

"We study the past to understand the present; we understand the present to guide the future."
—William Lund

In this book, my goal was to inform you about the role sugar has played in history and to shed light on how, through more healthy choices, a healthy lifestyle can be yours. Looking at sugar's role throughout history and up to the present day created a unique lens for me to view health epidemics that affect many Americans, especially people of color. The role of food, primarily sugar, has transformed the world as we currently know it, and it has had a major impact on the health of many civilizations. Sugar has been the one raw material that has consistently and constantly found itself at the forefront of any "modern" civilization's caloric intake. Currently, sugar and foods that quickly convert into sugar are still prevalent in our society and are wreaking havoc on our health, especially within lower socioeconomic communities. The same socioeconomic communities that are being ravaged by sugar are, typically, of the same ethnic groups that were enslaved by the sugar industry and brought to America via slavery. However, in today's modern society, those that are unaware of the impact of overconsumption of sugar and processed carbohydrates have all become enslaved by this one raw material.

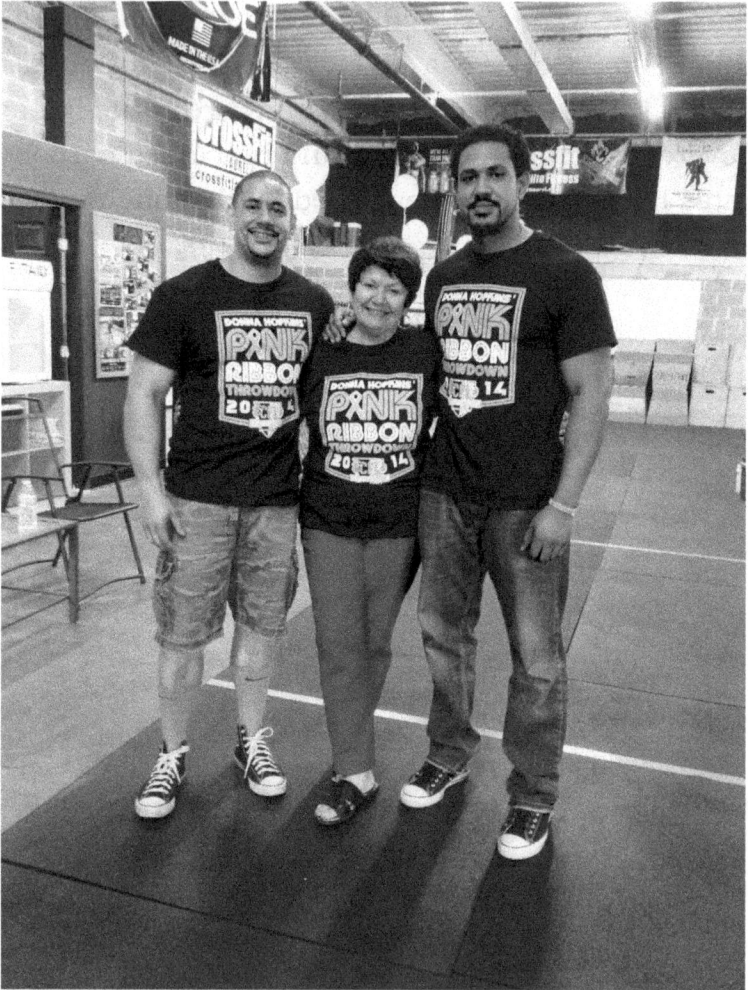

My mom and BIG lil bro during one of the many breast cancer fundraisers we've held.

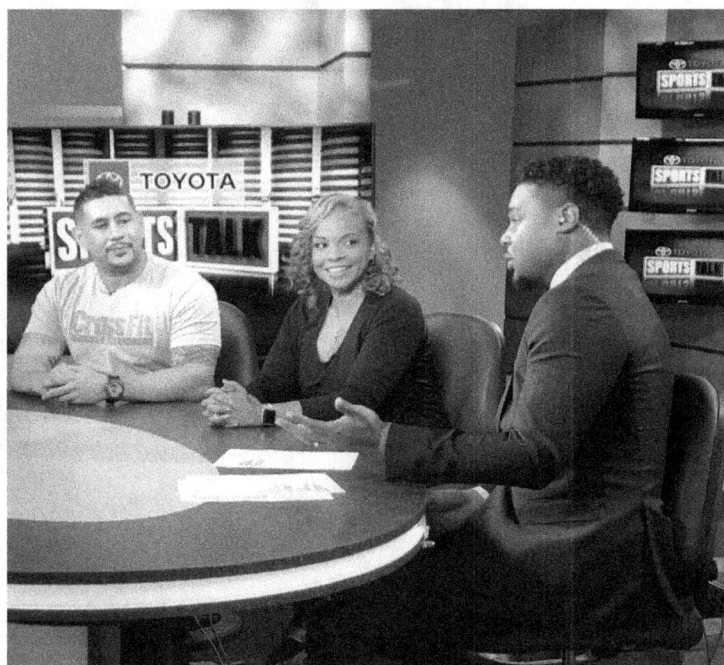

On the set of Sports Talk with my partner-in-health-and-fitness Mocha Lee along with host Robert Burton.

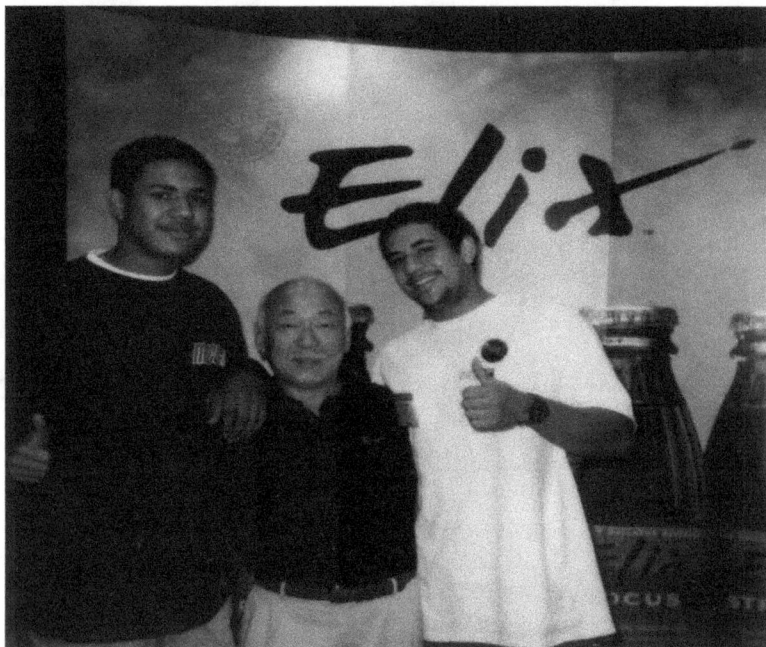

Me, my big little brother, and the one and only Pat Morita aka Mr. Miyagi! We were at one of the many Natural Products Expos we've attended and couldn't help but get a pic with the Karate Kid Master!

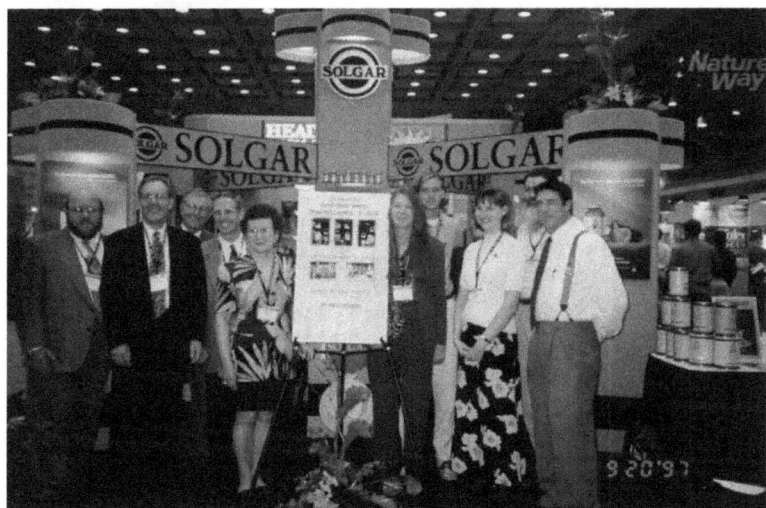

My grandparents had successfully expanded their health food store and this is a photo of my grandmother receiving an award for being the 2nd largest retailer in the COUNTRY for Solgar brand supplements.

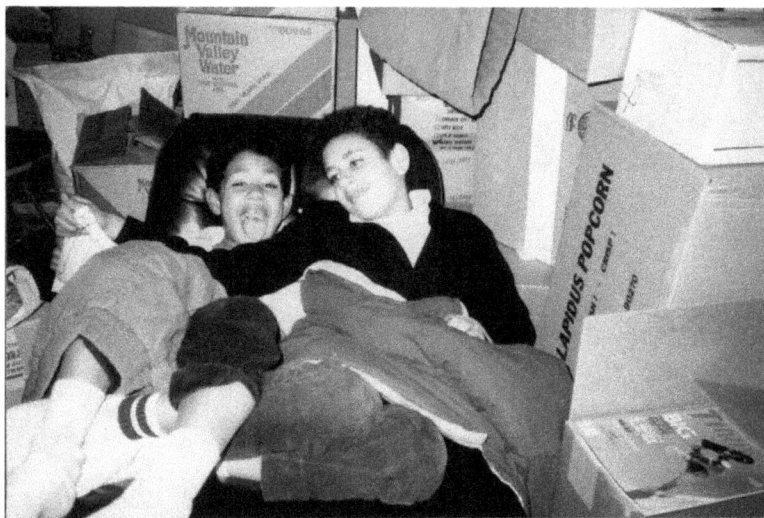

This is me and my little brother hanging out in the back room of Laurel Health Foods back in the early 80's. We did that almost every day and that old black recliner saw many naps. Check out the Mountain Valley Water boxes! I've been drinking "Alkaline" since the '80s! Also, check out the old-school "Thrasher" skateboard magazine!

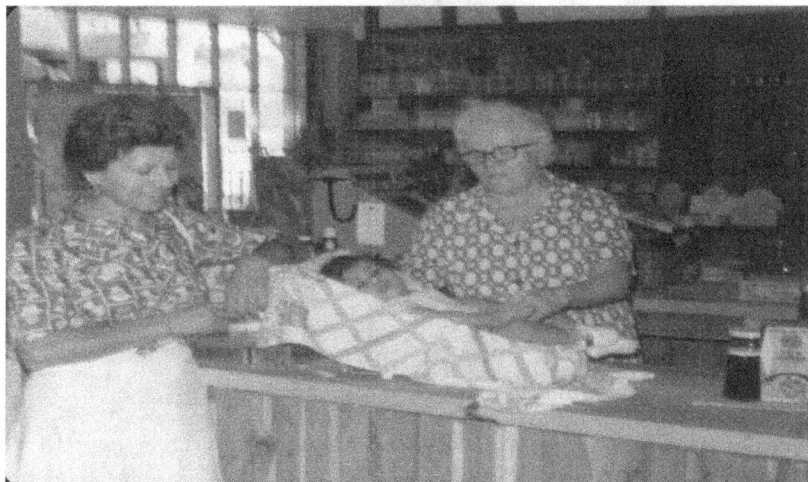

This is a picture of me lounging in my family's health food store like a little BOSS in 1976. The lady on the left is one of my grandmother's sisters, Aunt Annie, who was a big inspiration for my grandmother opening the health food store. The other lady is my great- grandmother aka Oma.

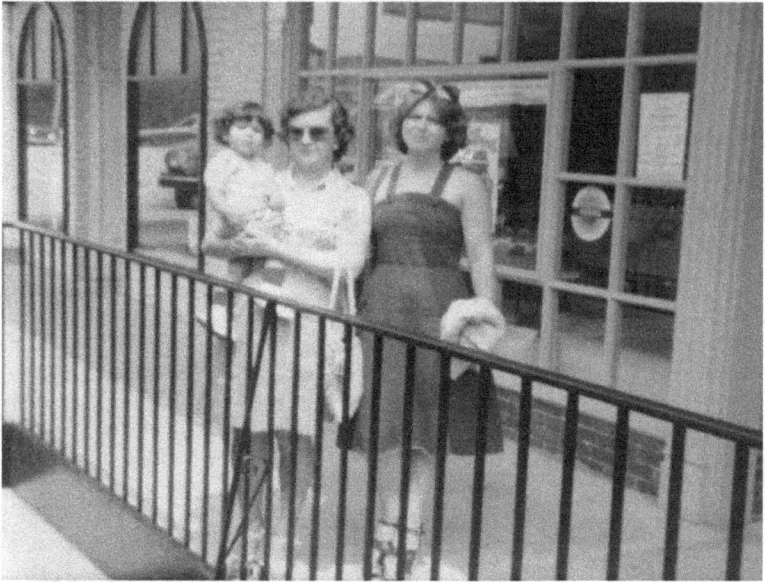

This is a 1970s throwback of me with my grand-mother and mom in front of the health food store.

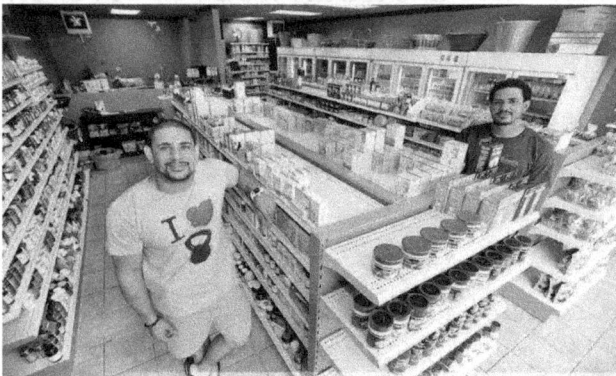

My brother and I when we moved the family health food store to Main St in Laurel, MD. At the time, it was the 5th move in Laurel Health Foods in its 44 years of being in business.

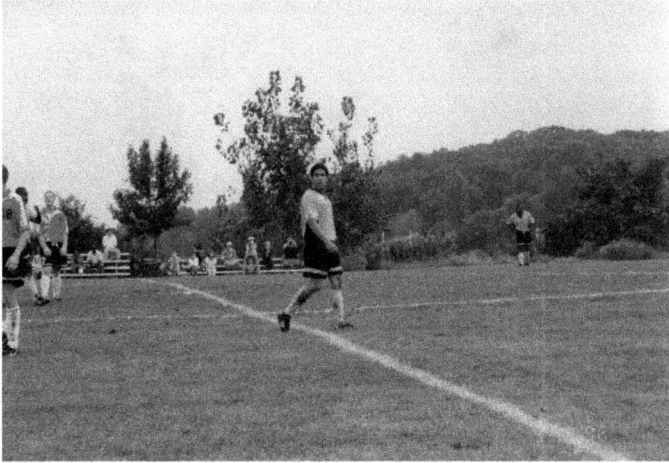

While attending Bowie State University, I played soccer and started paying attention to various sports supplements and spending more time in the weight room.

THANK YOU!

As we come to the end of this book, I would like to say, "Thank you!" First, thank you for supporting my dream of self-publishing my first book, and second, thank you for taking the time to read it! I hope you have found this book educational, informative, thought-provoking, and, at times, entertaining.

I would like to make a few special "Thank You's" to several people who have had an impact on my life as well as the formation of this book.

To my loving and supporting wife Paula, without you by my side, none of this would even have been possible! You always have my back and no matter how crazy my mind might be working you're there to support me. All the evenings when we pass each other like two ships in the night, you never stopped believing in my dream of not only finishing this book but all the other endeavors I've sought out. You are truly sent from heaven and you mean the world to me!

My two angels Laila and Aaron--having you in my life is a blessing beyond words. Watching you grow and learn in all aspects of life brings me joy every day! You are both amazing and growing up too fast. Laila has been promoting my book since she found about it several years ago, and I am happy to have her as my #1 hype girl! Of course, my best bud in the entire world Aaron aka Tom Cat ALWAYS has my back!

My mom and dad, Monika and Charles—you have always been in my corner and supported, well almost, all my wild and crazy ideas. You both have shown me the world and given me such a balanced life in such an unbalanced world.

My grandfather, Austin Lowe aka Pa, who sadly passed away in August 2022, who helped to fuel my imagination and taught me to not be afraid to dream. I am pretty sure that's where some of my wild and crazy ideas come from.

My big lil bro Phil, you've been in my corner from day one! Granted I did teach you how to walk but hey! You've been supportive of all those wild and crazy ideas over the years, and I am looking forward to the new ones that we are dreaming up. Can't stop, won't stop!

Dr. and Mrs. Shamim, you have no idea how much of an impact you have had on my life. Assisting your patients with purchasing the various supplements that you prescribed to them and to then see their health turn around was something beyond special. Thanks to you, I knew what candida was and how to pronounce acidophilus at a very young age. Although Dr. Shamim passed away during the editing of the 2nd edition of this book, he knew how much I appreciated his work ethic and approach to a healthy lifestyle.

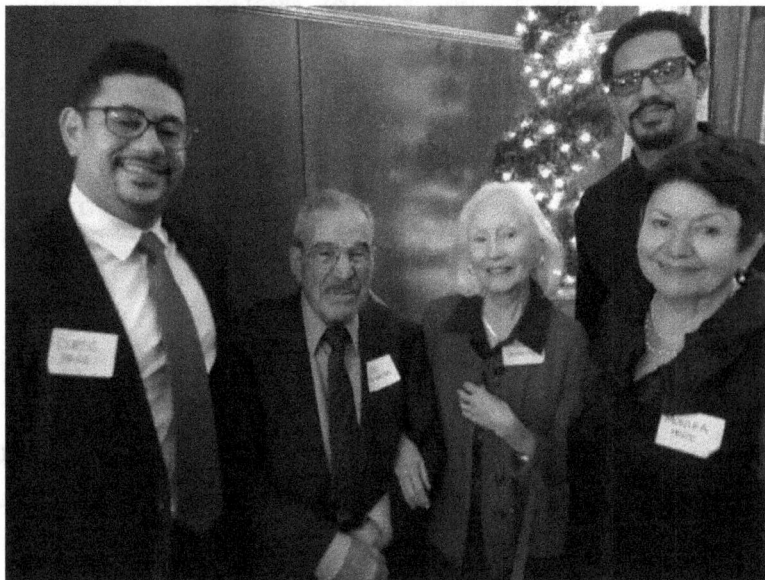

My mom, brother and me with Dr. and Mrs. Shamim at his 50 year of medical service celebration dinner.

Coach Robert Crawford, about 18 years ago I came into your boxing facility and my life has been changed ever since. Not only are you an amazing coach and teacher, but your kindness and love for teaching are a rare find. You didn't hesitate to let me coach folks in the back of your gym and on the many days nobody showed up, you'd just chuckle and tell me not to worry about it and to keep pushing forward.

Erica Riggio from Green Owl Designs—you took a leap of faith with this crazy gym I opened and have been a major supporter from day one. You were also there with me on many late nights helping to properly clean up this book and get it done! Your editing expertise, along with your support of what I wanted to put out, has been a true blessing.

Beverly Hunt—we reconnected while running into each other randomly at a local restaurant. That is when I mentioned this book to you that I had been working on and wanted to publish. We then spent many Friday nights at your dining room table taking what was a bunch of various concepts and writings and started to create this final product. Your belief in me and what I wanted to do helped serve as motivation to not give up and see it through.

To my dear Brenda Williams—you were one of my biggest cheerleaders and fans of this book. Your face would always light up when you'd tell me how you needed your copy signed. As the oldest athlete to train at Fraternal Elite Fitness, your commitment to getting healthy and losing weight was truly inspiring. Your tragic passing truly shook me to my core, and I know that you're looking down on me smiling. I hope that you've enjoyed the book and I have your signed copy set aside on my bookshelf.

To all the various athletes that have trusted me with their health and fitness over the years, thank you for entrusting me and my gym with your health and fitness. You only get one body and for you to come in and let me have the honor of assisting you with your health and wellness means a lot.

To the thousands of individuals that I have had the opportunity to meet via my family's health food store along with my own--allowing me to share my recommendations with you and assist with various questions has been an honor.

Last but definitely not least, I want to thank **YOU** for supporting me and purchasing this book. I also want to thank you for taking the time to actually read it and I hope that you were able to gain some knowledge from it.

Once again, THANK YOU!

And *cheers to Health, Wealth, and Prosperity!*

LET'S CONTINUE TO LEARN AND GROW TOGETHER

www.curtispricelive.com

www.theitisrevealed.com

www.fraternalfitness.com

Instagram: @curtispricelive

For booking speaking and workshop engagements please go to:

www.curtispricelive.com

MEET CURTIS

Curtis Price is passionate about inspiring others to live a healthy lifestyle. Health and wellness have been important aspects of his life from a very young age. His grandparents owned and operated one of the first health food stores on the East Coast and it has been a staple in the community since the 1970s. Spending the majority of his childhood around the store developed a unique perspective on the importance of food in a healthy lifestyle. This inspired him to open his own low-carb store called "Whoa..That's Lo!", which started off as a small section in his family's health food store. It soon expanded to two locations in the Maryland area and also gained national attention.

WHAT SETS CURTIS APART
FROM THE REST

- He has a very unique upbringing within the natural food industry
- He also pioneered opening one of the first low-carb stores in the country way before people knew what a carb was
- For the past 20 years, he has been helping people live a healthy lifestyle.
- He practices what he preaches
- He opened one of the first CrossFit Affiliates in the DC, Maryland, and Virginia area.
- Plus, he took a proactive look at sugar's role through history, how it fueled the slave trade to the Americas, how it is still enslaving people of color in America, and how you can break free from sugar's shackles

SPEAKING ENGAGEMENTS

- Sugar's Role Through History & How It Served As A Driving Force In Transporting Slaves To The Americas
- Look At The Modern Day Health Pandemic That Is Wreaking Havoc On Our Communities
- How You Can Once And For All Start Living A Healthy Lifestyle And Begin To Create Generational Health
- Take A Deep Dive Into The Book '*The Itis Revealed*" With Author Curtis Price

HEALTHY LIFESTYLE
DEVELOPMENT WORKSHOPS

- 4 Pillars of Health Workshop
- Flexitarian Living Blueprint Workshop

DIGITAL PRODUCTS

Book:

- *The Itis Revealed*

Online Courses:

- Zillion Dollar Math Course
- 4 Pillars of Health Master Class
- The 10 Healthy Lifestyle Commandments
- Stop Sabotaging Your Weight Loss

AFTERWORD

The first edition to *The Itis Revealed* was published in January 2020, (3 months before the COVID-19 pandemic lockdown). During the pandemic, I watched as so many health reports stated that the people who were succumbing to this disease at a faster rate were those with underlying health conditions. I sadly knew that people with obesity, diabetes and other pre-existing conditions were going to be one of the main groups to pass away from COVID-19. This inspired me even more to spread the word about the harmful health implications of having these issues. I went back through the book and changed the various graphs and charts into more attractive images hoping to grasp the readers attention. I also developed several courses that complement the book where I take a more personal and one on one approach to explaining the various tools and tips that I have successfully used for close to 30 years. In this post COVID-19 world, it is our responsibility to start to take our health and wellness into our own hands! I strongly encourage you to take the steps towards losing any excess weight and cutting out as much sugar and processed carbohydrates from your daily intake. The journey of one thousand miles ultimately begins with one step. I wish you nothing but the absolute best and know that I am with you cheering you on! I have complete faith in you as you work toward living a healthier, wealthier, and more prosperous life!

BIBLIOGRAPHY

Hello

1. (Mintz, 1986, p.32) Mintz, S. W. (1986). Sweet-ness and power: The place of sugar in modern history. Penguin p.32.

2. (Kaufmann & Holland, 2003, p. 25) Kaufmann, D. A. & Holland, D. (2003). Infectious diabetes: A cutting-edge approach to stopping one of America's fastest-growing epidemics in its tracks. Rockwall, Tex: Mediatrition p.25.

Chapter 1

1. ("SKIL – History of Sugar," 2018) SKIL – History of Sugar. (2018). Retrieved from http://www.sucrose.com/lhist.html
2. ("Slavery Timeline 1501–1600 – a Chronology of Slavery, Abolition, and Emancipation", 2018) Slavery Timeline 1501–1600 – a Chronology of Slavery, Abolition, and Emancipation. (2018). Retrieved from http://www.brycchancarey.com/slavery/chrono3.htm

3. ("Brazilian Independence | Boundless World History", 2018) Brazilian Independence | Boundless World History. (2018). Retrieved from https://courses.lumenlearning.com/boundless-worldhistory/chapter/brazilian-independence/
4. ("Plymouth Rock", 2018) Plymouth Rock. (2018). Retrieved from http://americanhistory.si.edu/press/fact-sheets/plymouth-rock
5. ("History", 2018) History. (2018). Retrieved from https://sweetsucrose.weebly.com/history.html
6. ("Digital History", 2018) Digital History. (2018). Retrieved from http://www.digitalhistory.uh.edu/disp_textbook.cfm?smtID=2&psid=3538
7. ("Act Prohibiting Importation of Slaves", 2018) Act Prohibiting Importation of Slaves. (2018). Retrieved from https://en.wikipedia.org/wiki/Act_Prohibiting_Importation_of_Slaves
8. (Amendment, 2018) Amendment, T. (2018). 13th Amendment – Black History – HISTORY.com. Retrieved from https://www.history.com/topics/black-history/thirteenth-amendment

9. ("SKIL – History of Sugar", 2018 SKIL – History of Sugar. (2018). Retrieved from http://www.sucrose.com/lhist.html

10.(Mintz, 1986, p.134) Mintz, S. W. (1986). Sweetness and Power: The Place of Sugar in Modern History. Penguin p.134

11.Mintz, S. (1986 [1985]) Sweetness and Power: The Place of Sugar in Modern History, London: Penguin. (p.134)

12.(Mintz, 1986, p.106) Mintz, S. W. (1986). Sweetness and Power: The Place of Sugar in Modern History. Penguin p.106

13.(Mintz, 1986, p.106) Mintz, S. W. (1986). Sweetness and Power: The Place of Sugar in Modern History. Penguin p.106

14.Faculty of Medicine, University of Bahr Elghazal.

15.(CITE). (https://www.diapedia.org/introduction-to-diabetes-mellitus/1104692125/aretaeus-of-cappadocia)

16.(Mintz, 1986, p.67) Mintz, S. W. (1986). Sweetness and Power: The Place of Sugar in Modern History. Penguin p.67

17.(Mintz, 1986, p.67) Mintz, S. W. (1986). Sweetness and Power: The Place of Sugar in Modern History. Penguin p.67

18. (Mintz, 1986, p.128) Mintz, S. W. (1986). Sweetness and Power: The Place of Sugar in Modern History. Penguin p.128
19. (Mintz, 1986, p.129) Mintz, S. W. (1986). Sweetness and Power: The Place of Sugar in Modern History. Penguin p.129
20. (Mintz, 1986, p.130) Mintz, S. W. (1986). Sweetness and Power: The Place of Sugar in Modern History. Penguin p.130

Chapter 2

1. (Vincenty, 2014)
2. (foodbycountry.com, 2018)
3. (LATIBAH Collard Green Museum, 2016)
4. (madehow.com, n.d.)
5. (foodbycountry.com, 2018)
6. (revolvy.com, n.d.)
7. (Olver, 2015)
8. (Dobsen, 2017)
9. (pulse.com.gh, 2015)
10. (Griot, 2017)
11. (blackthen.com, 2018)
12. (Sambira, 2018)
13. (Sambira, 2018)
14. ("Postprandial somnolence", 2018) Postprandial somnolence. (2018). Retrieved from https://en.wikipedia.org/wiki/Postprandial_s omnolence

15. ("List of medical roots, suffixes, and prefixes", 2018) List of medical roots, suffixes, and prefixes. (2018). Retrieved from <ins>https://en.wikipedia.org/wiki/List_of_medical_roots,_suffixes_and_prefixes</ins>

Chapter 3

1. ("Statistics about diabetes", 2018) Statistics about diabetes. (2018). Retrieved from http://www.diabetes.org/diabetes-basics/statistics/
2. ("Disease of the week – diabetes", 2018) Disease of the week – diabetes. (2018). Retrieved from https://www.cdc.gov/dotw/diabetes/index.html
3. (Association, 2018) Association, A. (2018). Latino Programs. Retrieved from http://www.diabetes.org/in-my-community/awareness-programs/latino-programs/
4. ("Statistics about diabetes", 2018) Statistics about diabetes. (2018). Retrieved from http://www.diabetes.org/diabetes-basics/statistics/
5. "Who are police killing?" *cjcj.org*. Center on Juvenile and Criminal Justice, n.d. Web. (1/7/2018)
6. (Association, 2018) Association, A. (2018). Latino Programs. Retrieved from

http://www.diabetes.org/in-my-community/awareness-programs/latino-programs/

7. ("Statistics about diabetes", 2018) Statistics about diabetes. (2018). Retrieved from http://www.diabetes.org/diabetes-basics/statistics/

Chapter 4

1. http://vegetarian.about.com/od/glos-sary/g/Vegan.htm
2. http://theveggietable.com/arti-cles/whatisavegetarian
3. ("What makes someone a vegan, and what do they eat, exactly?", 2018) What makes someone a vegan, and what do they eat, exactly? (2018). Retrieved from https://www.thespruceeats.com/what-do-ve-gans-eat-3376824
4. ("What is a vegetarian? – the veggie table", 2018) What is a vegetarian? – the veggie table. (2018). Retrieved from https://www.theveg-gietable.com/blog/vegetarianism/what-is-a-vegetarian/
5. ("Vegetarianism", 2018) Vegetarianism. (2018). Retrieved from https://en.wikipedia.org/wiki/Vegetarianism
6. http://en.wikipedia.org/wiki/vegetarianism)

7. ("Vegetarianism", 2018) Vegetarianism. (2018). Retrieved from https://en.wikipedia.org/wiki/Vegetarianism

Chapter 5

1. ("Glossary – organic.org", 2018) Glossary – organic.org. (2018). Retrieved from https://organic.org/glossary/
2. (Group, 2018) Group, E. (2018). EWG's 2018 shopper's guide to pesticides in produce. Retrieved from https://www.ewg.org/food-news/summary.php

Chapter 7

1. (Economic Significance of Mycotoxicoses. Pennington Center Nutrition Series. Vol. I: Mycotoxins, Cancer and Health. LSU Press. Baton Rouge. 1991.)
2. (Kaufmann, & Holland, 2003, p.34) Kaufmann, D. A., & Holland, D. (2003). Infectious diabetes: A cutting-edge approach to stopping one of America's fastest-growing epidemics in its tracks. Rockwall, Tex: Mediatrition p.34
3. ("*Candida albicans*", 2018) *Candida albicans*. (2018). Retrieved from https://en.wikipedia.org/wiki/Candida_albicans
4. (Kaufmann, & Holland, 2003, p.32) Kaufmann, D. A., & Holland, D. (2003). Infectious diabetes:

A cutting-edge approach to stopping one of America's fastest-growing epidemics in its tracks. Rockwall, Tex: Mediatrition p.32

5. ("Trading Alcoholism for Sugar Addiction: The Not-So-Sweet Truth," 2018) Trading Alcoholism for Sugar Addiction: The Not-So-Sweet Truth. (2018). Retrieved from https://www.promises.com/articles/alcohola buse/trading-alcoholism-for-sugar-addiction/

6. (Kaufmann, & Holland, 2003, p.178) Kaufmann, D. A., & Holland, D. (2003). Infectious diabetes: A cutting-edge approach to stopping one of America's fastest-growing epidemics in its tracks. Rockwall, Tex: Mediatrition. P.178

7. ("Jarisch-Herxheimer reaction", 2018) Jarisch–Herxheimer reaction. (2018). Retrieved from https://en.wikipedia.org/wiki/Jarisch%E2%8 0%93Herxheimer_reaction

Chapter 8

1. ("Type 1 Diabetes", 2018) Type 1 Diabetes. (2018). Retrieved from http://www.diabetes.org/diabetes-basics/type-1/?loc=db-slabnav

2. ("Type 1 Diabetes", 2018) Type 1 Diabetes. (2018). Retrieved from http://www.diabetes.org/diabetes-basics/type-1/?loc=db-slabnav.

3. ("2003 Words of the Year American Dialect Society", 2004) 2003 Words of the Year American Dialect Society. (2004). Retrieved from
https://www.americandialect.org/2003_word s_of_the_year
4. (Pescatore, 2004, p.32) Pescatore, F. (2004). The Hamptons Diet: Diet secrets of the rich, famous and thin. John Wiley & Sons p.32
5. (Pescatore, 2004, p.33) Pescatore, F. (2004). The Hamptons Diet: Diet secrets of the rich, famous and thin. John Wiley & Sons p.33
6. (Pescatore, 2004, p.34) Pescatore, F. (2004). The Hamptons Diet: Diet secrets of the rich, famous and thin. John Wiley & Sons p.34
7. Wikipedia contributors. (2019, December 16). Sugar substitute. In *Wikipedia, The Free Encyclopedia*. Retrieved 14:43, December 19, 2019, from
https://en.wikipedia.org/w/index.php?ti-tle=Sugar_substitute&oldid=931085438

www.ingramcontent.com/pod-product-compliance
Lightning Source LLC
Chambersburg PA
CBHW061746270326
41928CB00011B/2394